Tour of Duty

Tour of Duty

50 Inspiring Stories from Our Men and Women in the Armed Forces

Lynne Marie Rominger and Milo James

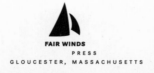

FAIR WINDS
PRESS
GLOUCESTER, MASSACHUSETTS

Text © 2003 by Lynne Marie Rominger and Milo James

First published in the U.S.A. by

Fair Winds Press
33 Commercial Street
Gloucester, Massachusetts 01930-5089

Library of Congress Cataloging-in-Publication Data available

10 9 8 7 6 5 4 3 2

ISBN 1-59233-012-6

Cover design by Mary Ann Smith
Design by Laura Herrmann Design

Printed and bound in Canada

To the guardians of the flame, and especially those who have paid the ultimate price, may their memories be eternal.

Contents

Introduction

We, authors of *Tour of Duty*, one a U.S. Army veteran and each from a proud heritage of military service, conceived this project out of a desire to familiarize Americans with those who serve and have served our great Republic in uniform. Without them, even the freedom to write or read this book would, quite literally, be no more than an unrealized or, perhaps worse, forgotten principle.

Herein, we have painted with a broad brush a picture of the face of the man or woman in uniform, revealing both the universality and diversity of military service and, it is hoped, edifying those currently serving with the knowledge that the country supports them. Military service, fundamentally, is as unique as each person wearing the uniform; yet, there is a commonality in military service, regardless of branch, rank, gender, or race. It is challenging to describe the ethos among those who have in common the matchless experience of military life. It is perhaps better to convey, however imperfectly, through personal accounts a sense of the esprit de corps in military men and women that inspires camaraderie, courage, devotion, humor, spirituality, and an unwavering solicitude for the honor of the group.

Between the covers of this unpretentious book, fifty true vignettes present real men and women who sacrificed of themselves for us. No branch of service is favored, no time period preferred. These stories reveal ordinary Americans in extraordinary circumstances, from the mountains of Afghanistan to the beaches of Normandy, from sultry jungles to the Arctic Circle, from the seas to the sky. We will confront the horror of war and venerate the unfathomable fortitude of those embroiled in it, laugh at the creative wit engendered by camaraderie, salute honor born out of self-sacrifice, cheer the liberation of prisoners of war, and praise the achievement of childhood dreams. *Esprit de corps*, a term whose meaning is inculcated in every recruit from the first day of boot camp or basic training, is to the military what a catalyst is to a chemical reaction, and silently grows powerful in the hearts of men and women during their widely disparate tours of duty.

Many stories resulted from personal interviews conducted over lunch, over scotch and cigars, or simply over the telephone. Others the subjects personally wrote. Perhaps most compelling, however, are those oral histories compiled by a group of stellar high school students from a National Blue Ribbon High School.

Encouraged to "raise the bar," the students, embracing the assignment, overwhelmingly exceeded expectations. They interviewed family members, friends, and neighbors, and wrote superlative historical accounts of their subjects' tours of duty. All discovered ideals like camaraderie, honor, and heroism; many found within their own families legacies of patriotism and sacrifice they never knew existed. Ultimately, however, they learned that, although the soldier is the last to want to fight, he or she is the first willing to fight for the freedom and security we all enjoy.

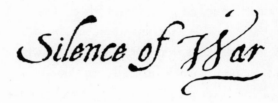

Silence of War

By Warren G. Harding

as told by his granddaughter, Caitlin Culbertson

It all happened so very fast. It was a beautiful feeling to be on the shores of Hawaii. The scents of flowers and palm trees mixed with the gust of the fresh morning breezes. It seemed like a normal Pearl Harbor morning, a morning where nothing could go wrong, a morning just like the rest. But I was wrong.

As I stepped out onto the deck of our ship, the USS *California*, I wondered how long Frank would be. He was to join me for lunch that day at the home of old friends, the Hiram Miles family, in Honolulu. Frank wasted a lot of time that morning; he was drinking coffee with one hand and dressing with the other.

"Come on. Get going!" I yelled.

"The prospect of spending a whole day with someone I don't know is not exciting enough for me to hurry anything. Certainly one lunch doesn't matter," he replied.

As I turned to walk away, he yelled, "Go ahead on. I'll be out in a minute. If we miss the 0730, we'll catch the 0800. That will get us to Fleet Landing in time to meet your friend from the *Arizona*."

I walked out to where the officer of the day was standing near the gangway. As I looked down I saw the 0730 pull away. "Gosh nab it,

Frank!" I yelled. The feeling of extreme madness consumed me for but a minute, for the smell of fresh bread and gardenias filled my nose once again. That smell always brought a peaceful feeling to me. What a time to be alive, young, and ready for anything coming my way!

Nearly a half hour had passed from when I first started watching the morning activities. Wondering where in the hell Frank was, I started to watch the band form for colors. That's when I first heard it—a sound so unmistakable it chills my blood to remember it. Looking up, I saw the diving plane heading straight for the Ford Island airstrip. As it sped steadily downward, the Japanese plane with the knife-pointed wings appeared to stop dead in the air for a moment, as if to survey for one second what was before him.

The bomb fell. It exploded on the runway. I could not see it for the guns were in my way. But I could hear it, and I could feel it. The debris flew all over, even out beyond my ship. A band from another ship started to play colors. Another bomb fell, this time closer to our ship. Dave Kennedy, the assistant bandmaster, saw the explosions and dismissed the *California* band to battle stations. A signalman tried to secure colors to the jack but he didn't make it. The *California* fought through the entire conflict without colors in place.

I stopped only for a moment to take it all in and look about for Frank one more time. Then I headed for my battle station. Over the intercom I could hear a marine shouting in an excited voice, "Battle Stations! Battle Stations! General Quarters! General Quarters! General Quarters! This is no shit. We're at war!"

Down one ladder, then two, then three, and I was there, the first one actually. So, I grabbed the headphones and the microphone and waited for the others to arrive. Surprisingly enough, the entire repair party of fourteen men, including me and the chief shipfitter, assembled within a few short minutes.

The chief made sure we were all accounted for, then he secured us in. We were committed. No beds, no food, no water. Just metal walls and airtight secured doors, and thirteen other men whom we barely knew, all sealed in a small underwater compartment.

Central communications had asked for a report and I spoke into the microphone, "Repair four port all present and accounted for, sir."

"Repair four port, aye, stand by for further orders."

"Repair four port, aye."

Then it happened—we were hit. We could feel the heated metal bending and re-forming. We slipped and spun as the water and oil leaked through the very small holes that watertight compartment allowed. The sound of men dying and the screaming of the wounded and the groan of the ship as it started to sink to the harbor mud filled our ears and minds. Then it stopped.

Just as fast as the sounds had ceased, they began again. Screams and cries and loud booms were all over. A leak began to form in an aft watertight door. We watched it form a small puddle on the ground. The hole was about as big as the mouth of a water bottle. Without hesitation, the chief checked the compartment next to ours for free space. When he realized it was free, he loosened the levers and swung the metal door open and we all moved forward.

The first thing I noticed about this new compartment was that there was no ladder to the topside; there was only an ammunition conveyer belt and a wind shaft that reached all the way up to the boat deck. The wind shaft looked large enough to hold a small person. I leaned over the conveyer belt to look up the shaft and a flush of fresh air hit my face; it felt good.

We were wet but comfortable. We prayed the ship would not turn on its side, because the shaft would fill with water and we would all be goners. But for the time being, we had fresh air and plenty of it. All we could do was wait. Nearly five minutes later I reported to central communications with our new location. They responded with, "Repair four port, and all stations, the ship is damaged. We caught a torpedo hit aft launched by low flying aircraft. We're at war and sinking. Some are going over the side. Planes are strafing from the port side. The *Casson* and the *Downs* just blew up. The Wee Vee"—the USS *West Virginia*—"is on fire. And the *Nevada* is getting under way. They're in the channel and headed for open sea. Oh, my God! The *Arizona* just blew sky high! It broke in the middle like a monster firecracker. Smoke and fire is a mile in the air.

"No ammunition when we finally got permission to open the locked ready boxes! We're forming an ammunition working party all the way down the midships hatch right into the magazine. Gotta get some antiaircraft shells to fight these yellow bastards!

"Have nothing to fight with! Some of the guys are so pissed off, they broke in the spud locker. Now they're throwing potatoes at planes flying near enough to crash into us!

"This is horrible!

"Lordy mercy! One of our men just dived out of the sky lookout fifty feet above us. He did a perfect Olympic swan dive. WOW! He made it. There he is. He surfaced. A small barge is picking him up. What a dive!

"They strafed our own liberty launch in the open channel. The cox'n tried to change direction from Fleet Landing, to make a hurried return to the ship. He didn't make it. It looks like all hands died in the launch. Some are hanging over the side with their head and shoulders dragging in the water.

"All guys sealed in, stand by! We cannot break watertight integrity. The ship is hanging by the hawsers. Damage control is going to see if they can do some counter flooding to keep the ship from capsizing. Out."

"Wait, don't go," I thought. That's the launch Frank and I missed. "Four port, aye, aye," was all I could get out.

More explosions resounded. A double hit picked the ship up and settled it back down at a fifteen-degree position. The battleship *California* sank to the quarterdeck with me in it. Buried alive with thirteen other comrades and no way out. "Are we going to die here?" someone asked.

"Hard to tell, Mac, we may be here awhile," was all the chief could say.

Hit after hit, they just kept coming. We just sat back and prayed for the lives we could hear being taken away. Trapped in a compartment, our ears and minds open to the sounds of chilling screams and death-ly cries, there was nothing else we could do. Then suddenly—it seemed like hours later—the voice from central communications came back on. But what we thought would bring relief only brought more terror. "All hands abandon ship! Abandon ship! Repair four port, remain. Repeat, remain. Do not, repeat, do not break watertight integrity. We'll be back when we can reboard the ship."

Chills went up my spine, around my neck, down my stomach, and to my toes, where they stopped. The words *abandon ship* iced my bones. I looked down to see a mixture of water and oil that had begun to gather around my newly pressed white bell-bottoms.

Being the only one with a headset, I alone knew the orders. I was uneasy with my secret but kept it to myself. I reported back to central for a confirmation. "That is confirmed, I am leaving now," I heard the voice on the other end say. Then there was a click and deathly silence followed. All eyes were on me. I told them that central was moving their position. I didn't want to lie, but the thought of everyone know-ing they couldn't save themselves was worse than just one holding it in himself.

Silence suddenly enveloped the little room. Then, after a few minutes, a bomb exploded in the midships hatch above us, and it was every man for himself. Bracketed by three torpedoes—one aft, two for-ward—while a five hundred–pound bomb burst above us, it seemed hopeless. More explosions, and the watertight seal on the door broke. A mixture of fuel, oil, and water seeped through. The smell and feel were awful. The compartment floor became very slippery. We found a monkey wrench under the conveyer belt and tried to fix the hole, but it was no use. Though the hole wasn't huge, it was large enough that it would soon allow our small compartment to fill.

Silence again, even weightier than before. A shipfitter found a gui-tar and started strumming notes to "You Are My Sunshine." We all sang along for a couple of lines, then just stopped, realizing we might never see the sunlight again. No one said a word; the singing just stopped. Several hours passed, and nothing was said. The only sound was that of our swishing and sliding through the oil and fuel as we moved about the compartment.

By noon, there were no more sounds of battle. No more anxiety, just the thoughts that ran through our minds. Someone finally broke the silence. "There is water and oil in the compartment behind us, there is water and oil forward. There isn't much we can do, is there?" He didn't speak directly to anyone, and no one responded. We just sat there and thought about what he had said.

When Chips, a carpenter, started to write on a bulkhead, we turned to watch. "What's that all about?"

"I'm writing my will," Chips said. "I'm writing how I want my part of the farm back home shared with my brother and sisters."

Soon others began writing their wills on the bulkhead also. After some thought, since I owned nothing but my trombone, I figured why not scrawl a simple letter on the bulkhead:

Dear Jack,

Some day when they raise the ole Prune Barge, someone will read this message to you, you will hear about it. The fact that we are writing our wills will be sensational enough to cause someone to get the message to you. You are only nine years old now; but you will read about what happened here for years to come. Learn not to trust the Japanese. They bombed us without warning, and though I may never see daylight, except through the wind shaft in this compartment, I want you to know that someone betrayed us. We believe Washington knew this was about to happen, and allowed it. . . .to get us involved.

We sighted subs last week, and last night the void spaces throughout the Fleet were ordered open overnight. . . . Never before in the history of the Navy has that happened. Our ship is still afloat with a heavy port list, and we will probably capsize unless someone does some fancy counter flooding. Our hawsers won't be able to hold us much longer.

I want you to have my little black book, if someone ever finds it. Right now it's in my locker on the main deck. The key to the locker is in my pocket. Write to those who appear with addresses. The others are not important. My trombone is in its case under my bunk in the Band quarters. It should survive this hellfire. If it does, I want you to have it.

Remember, my last thoughts were for you, Janie, Junie, and Mother and Pop.

The Navy is a good place to be. I wish I could have enjoyed it more. In the wrong place at the wrong time I guess.

If you ever get into a spot like this, just keep saying your name to yourself, as I am saying my name now. Say "My name is Jack Harding, and I fear no other. My name is Jack Harding, and I fear no other."

Signed,
Warren G. Harding

We wrote and read only our own wills. There was an unspoken privacy that kept us from looking at each other's. There was a strong feeling of emotion and respect that now came over our crew. Thoughts consumed our minds; these thoughts were private and self-contained. Perhaps we were unwilling to admit we were about to die, but whatever it was, we were comfortable with each other.

One of the small shoplifters whom we nicknamed "Shorty" jumped onto the conveyer belt and looked straight up the shaft into the sky and looked back at us and began to smile. The chief looked at him with a look of discontent and asked, "What's so damned funny?"

"Chief, you are not going to believe this but I can get out of here!"

"You can what? How do you think you are going to do that little miracle?"

"Fear not, I can climb that wind shaft and get out on the boat deck."

"But we've got to stay here," someone said.

"That's true, but there is an 'abandon ship' order also," I quietly said.

All eyes were now set on me.

"Abandon ship?"

"When did they abandon ship?"

"A long time ago," I said

"Why didn't you tell us? We could have been out there!"

"Where you gonna go?" I asked defensively.

Looking at each other for a definitive answer, they began to smile. The idea that I kept that information to myself for over five hours so as not to panic them, astonished them. Forgiveness flushed their souls of any harsh feelings.

"So how about it, Chief?" Shorty interrupted. "May I get permission to inch up that chute and see about finding a way to get you guys out?"

"Well?" the chief said, while looking to us for a response.

"Sure, Chief, let him go. The worst that can happen, he won't make it and end up back down here with us again."

"Right you are, Chief."

"Make it your best shot, Shorty," the chief ordered.

"Go ahead on."

Shorty started to get ready for his trip up the chute. The chief commented that he should strip to his undershorts to get a better grip. Another commented that he should take his shoes and socks off also. As he stripped to his undergarments, we all held our breath hoping the plan would work. He jumped onto the conveyer belt and started to inch his way up the shoot. His small little body fit easily into the space, with room to spare. He yelled that the metal was freezing. We told him to save his breath and use the energy to get up the chute. Higher and higher he inched, cussing, yelling, scraping, and slamming. We could hear him slip over the metal as if it were a falling-down ladder. But that didn't stop him.

"One more foot and I'll be there," he yelled down to us. "I made it! I made it!" he screamed with joy. "But I can't get out. There is a screen here to keep anyone from throwing garbage in the shaft. It keeps garbage out; but it keeps me in. A lot like fences."

The chief jumped on the conveyer belt and with no hesitation stuck his head in the shaft and yelled with all his might, "Kick the sonuvabitch out with your feet!"

"Okay, Chief! You got it!"

We could hear the kicking and scraping and pushing and shoving and the rattle, yet nothing. He said to us with a tired voice, "I can't get it." We screamed at him to keep trying. Finally, he broke the screen, tore it free, and jumped out.

"I'm out fellers, and I'll be back. I'm on my way, Chief. You guys hang on down there, and I'll find a work party to get you out. Maybe we can pump the water out of the other compartment or sumthin'."

His voice trailed off as we heard him say, "Lord help 'em." Then the footsteps faded away.

"Okay, kid," the chief hollered back. "Go get 'em!"

Faces and spirits changed quickly. Smiles filled the room. Our spirits were high and our hopes even higher. Now, we just had to sit back and wait—perhaps the hardest thing we had done so far.

I repeatedly said my name to myself as I had told my brother to do in my letter. Then I prayed, "Lord God of the universe, make it possible for me to get out of this can I'm in and give me a chance to be a man with a woman, any woman—clean, friendly, and willing to abide my inexperience long enough for me to learn something. I'm too young to die without having at least one chance to make love." The realization that I might die a virgin hit me and hit me hard. I wasn't ready to die. I didn't want to go yet. These thoughts just made me pray harder for Shorty's return.

"It's three o'clock," said the chief.

"I wonder how Shorty is doin'."

Unexpectedly, a tapping echoed in our little chamber.

"Is that you tapping on the bulkhead, Red?"

TAP, TAP, TAP.

"No, I thought it was you, Chief."

Over and again the tapping sounded the bulkhead. We grabbed a dog wrench and headed for the compartment door, the one we assumed kept us safe from a deluge pressing on the other side. The chief rammed open the door and there was Shorty on the other side, with water and oil now up to his waist. All bloody and scratched, he was a sight for sore eyes. The chief nearly tackled him with excitement.

"You little bastard, you did it!"

"Is it clear topside?" we asked.

"Yeah it's clear, but you don't want to see it. From here on it gets bad. The Fleet is in flames. We are in flames. There are bodies dead and still dying. There is an awful mess around the midships hatch. That must have been the last explosion we heard this morning. The ship is listing hard to port. Water is over the quarterdeck and half the port side of the fantail. Colors are nowhere in sight."

"Have the Japs stopped bombing? Is it safe to go on up and out?"

"Sure but watch where you walk. You may be stepping on the innards of one of your shipmates."

I was the last to leave the compartment that day. I gently laid the headphones on top of the conveyer belt and sighed with relief. I slipped and stumbled over to the next room, looking back but once to think about the time that I had spent in the room that day. I glanced up at the bulkhead where I had written my will and where the others had left theirs. There was no use for them anymore, but there was no reason to go back and erase them. Someone will read them someday when the old ship is raised and realize how seven hours trapped in a steel cage can transform boys into men.

•••

BIOGRAPHY: *Warren G. Harding was born in 1921 in New Point, Indiana. At the age of eighteen, Harding enlisted in the U.S. Navy. After World War II, Warren attended Wabash, worked in Washington, D.C., as a code breaker, and later pursued a successful career in real estate. Warren G. Harding died in San Jose, California, at the age of seventy-seven.*

A Special Force

BY JOHN DUNCAN

T here was one reason I joined the military—to become a spy, a special operator. I wanted to serve but also to mix it with adventure, action, and truly do something for the "good guys." Real life is different from boyish aspiration, so I did get to serve but did not get the career path that would lead to special operations. I was, however, fortunate to serve very closely with special operations men in several places, most interestingly in Haiti during our nation's activities there in the mid-1990s.

What I saw in Haiti in small ways had confirmed the big truths that I had always known. These were real men, true heroes with whom we have recently become reacquainted as a nation, men with character and deep concern for their fellow men, men of intellect and keen physical ability. These were the special operators that I had wanted to be.

No one knew how the mission in Haiti would develop. Fortunately for me, my workspace was collocated with the supporting contingent of Special Forces soldiers. They were present in Haiti for their skills in working with foreign cultures, building relationships with local people, teaching and training, and caring for peoples in the most basic areas of nutrition, hygiene, governance, and much more.

They were also present for their expert understanding of the dangers and methods of nefarious and "bad" people, and how to expertly deal with them in these far-flung areas of the world.

It was easy, I am sure, for them to see my enthusiasm for what they had done on their missions in one or another part of the world. They were kind to share their experiences during the typically slow times at the base camp. Their demeanor spoke clearly of their maturity, skill, and poise. As I heard their stories and saw them work, I was struck by the thought, "They do it!" You know the "it" I am speaking about? It is the "it" that is: parachuting, scuba diving, shooting all the weapons, building things, breaking things, speaking foreign languages in danger- ous places, making it happen, whatever "it" had to be. Just to go through my mundane tasks near them was a private joy.

All of them were friendly and carried themselves with natural and confident openness. I got to work with several of these guys on a reg- ular basis as part of my duties—from their commander, Major Fox, to a regular guy, their unit's workhorse, Sergeant King. There were two captains in particular who included me in as much as they could, Mitch Wilcox and Chris Gottschalk. I have worked with many talent- ed, extremely dedicated people all throughout the military and beyond. These guys, though, were the all-stars, at the top of their "game." They actually did what they trained for and did "it" every day, not three or four times in a career. And whatever they did, they did it well.

Both Chris and Mitch could have played any one of several pro- fessional sports. Mitch was the tallest man in the compound (perhaps in the country) and looked like an NFL linebacker. Chris could have been the opposing team's tight end. These two could as easily have been successful attorneys, doctors, or diplomats, and, in a very real way, they were all of these things. Mitch's may have been the harder, but both came from average or typical American backgrounds. These were ordinary men whom the United States allowed to serve us all in extraordinary ways.

As the military operation unfolded in Haiti, everything showed how oppressed the people had been, not only by their corrupt leadership but also by their wretched circumstances. It was clear that these desperate people could not mount any kind of resistance and clearly did not want to do so. Mitch and Chris routinely traveled to the remote parts of our area to meet these people and address their many needs. They even officially included me on a few of these patrols in our immediate area. This was something of a bureaucratic miracle, for an intelligence staff weenie assigned to the straightlaced and severe light infantry to accompany the easygoing, not always by the book, but always effective Special Forces.

Not every patrol was official. On one of the "unofficial" patrols, I was able to see a snapshot of what made these forces, well, so "special."

One evening the local Haitians were able to celebrate one of their annual holidays for the first time in several years. Mitch swung by my makeshift office to invite me on his patrol. This was the closest that I would ever get, so I made the most of it. Frankly, it was more danger-ous to stroll in the towns outside some of our forts in the United States. We walked along a wide street on the edge of town. It was empty, as most of the residents were at the city center for the revelry. Mitch and I chatted with the townspeople as we made our way through the city—a lady who sold fried bread, the local television repairman (since U.S. forces restored power, he had a surge in demand for his skills), and the casual passerby. Mitch knew some French, some Creole, and a lot about people. Each conversation was a mix of personal inter-est and strategic diplomacy.

And there were always unexpected, odd sights in Haiti. It was a country with one foot in the Stone Age and one in the modern age. One such sight that evening was a man and his family riding on a moped—his wife was seated behind him, one child stood on the foot rest to the side, another was sidesaddle on a basket over the rear tire, the third on the handlebars, feet dangling over the front tire. Each of them was carrying a portion of the family's belongings. It might have been a circus act in another part of the world. Mitch and I watched as this family circled around toward us to follow the road out of town.

Much had been neglected in Haiti, too. There were no streetlights, no meaningful road maintenance, and no civic support of any kind. The odd "circus family" scene took an unexpected, tragic turn when the moped dropped from sight—family, belongings, and all. The road had given way to a large sinkhole. The force of the small cycle's crash sent the littlest child careening from the handlebars into the curbside. From where I stood, fairly close by, I watched the pavement peel back the skin from his tiny forehead. To this day, the image is a flash of white quickly covered by red from blood. In my short time in Haiti, I had seen minor events like this flare into knots of violence and mob mania. I turned quickly to follow Mitch's lead but suddenly could not find him in the unlit, tropical night. As quickly as I could utter "Mitch," he spoke, directing me to watch the road toward town, not for mobs necessarily, but for other vehicles. His voice had come from the sinkhole. In the flash of time that it took for fear and adrenaline to rise in me, he had already moved into the sinkhole to render aid. I moved into the road to gain a better vantage and was able to glimpse what Mitch was doing. In a land rife with medieval maladies and modern epidemics, including widespread HIV, this professional was rendering first aid to the very bloody tiny boy. Mitch wore no gloves and fairly embraced the child as he applied disinfectant and bandages. In the moments that it took for this scene to develop, Mitch had not only assessed and bandaged the boy, but he had moved the child's mother to the roadside so that she could have an unobstructed view of Mitch removing the entire family and their belongings from the sinkhole, and radioing ahead to the aid station on behalf of this family in need. He did it all smoothly, calmly, engaging each of these people in the most constructive way. We then resumed our patrol through the otherwise festive city, meeting and speaking with many other people, continuing business as usual in this unusual place.

What was to me one of the most profound moments in my life was only a minor deed for Mitch, for Chris, for Sergeant King, and for those like them. These are the professionals who represent the very best in the profession of arms, our country, and all of us. By no means are they the only ones, these men at the forefront of service. I am moved when I read of the actions of men like these, seeking adventure, seeking to do what is right, seeking most of all to serve. Occasionally and always tragically, a story of their deeds is recognized with a medal or in the media. These profound acts of heroism are simple acts of service. There are so many acts that are not recognized in this life, but these simple acts of service are a part of every day in these men's careers.

•••

BIOGRAPHY: *John Duncan was born in San Benito, Texas. He attended the United States Military Academy, West Point, New York. On active duty John was stationed in Arizona and New York and served with the 10th Mountain Division at Fort Drum. He also served in the U.S. Army Reserve in California and New Jersey. Currently, John is a full-time civilian living with his wife and three children in New Jersey.*

Aim High

By Captain John Antedomenico, USAF

as told to Milo James

During grade school, my neighbor, a World War II instructor pilot, owned a single-engine Cessna 172. Knowing my interest in flying, one New Year's Day, to my great pleasure, he took my dad and me up in his plane. Safely airborne, without objection from Dad, I took the controls and flew a few exhilarating—though to Dad, slightly stomach-churning—maneuvers. Thrilled, I began that day to think about a career in the Air Force. In high school, due in large part to my mom's persistence, I applied to the Air Force Academy, despite my guidance counselor's discouragement; she actually told me, due to my average performance in high school, I should not waste my time applying.

Far from having wasted my time, however, I was accepted and, after graduating, went to the 640th Air Mobility Support Squadron at Howard Air Force Base in Panama. As a transportation officer, I supervised cargo and passenger loading operations, primarily in connection with resupplying embassies, radar facilities, and other U.S. assets in Latin America and the Caribbean. While I enjoyed my job, my childhood dream of flying never waned. One sultry Central American afternoon during some downtime, I took a break outside the aerial port to ponder my career opportunities. On the one hand, I truly liked my job; on the other, however, my dream still tugged at my heart.

While I sat there thinking (and sweating) in the torrid jungle heat, I watched a flight of F-15 Eagles from a Hawaii Air National Guard unit take off on some drug-interdiction-related mission. With unimaginable speed and an enveloping roar that rocked the entire base, one by one, the $30-million fighter jets shot down the runway, lifting into the air with a grace that belied their ferocity. Thrusting skyward at an angle and speed unlike any commercial aircraft, the F-15s' afterburners punctuated the twin turbofan engines with two fiery twelve-foot tongues. Transfixed, in that moment I became the little boy in the Cessna once again; I had to fly.

In 1999, after completing flight training at Whiting Field (NAS Pensacola), Vance Air Force Base, Randolph Air Force Base, and Tyndall Air Force Base, I joined the 58th Fighter Squadron (the "Gorillas"), 33d Fighter Wing. I'd been with the Gorillas about ten months when we received orders to Saudi Arabia in support of Operation Southern Watch to monitor and control the Iraqi skies south of the 33rd parallel. As part of the advanced echelon team, I arrived in-country a couple of weeks prior to the rest of my squadron. As a result, I was the first wingman in the squadron to fly a combat mission over Iraq. On that particular day, there was significant activity near the No-Fly Zone by Iraqi MiG-25 Foxbats—Soviet-era interceptors flown by the Iraqi air forces. Since I'd never done a combat mission before this, just the thought of getting up there was enough to get my blood going. I was to fly as a wingman, subordinate to my flight lead. Before we took off, he told me, "Just stay visual with me, Jack, and you'll be fine."

Sitting alone in my cockpit—the McDonnell Douglas F-15C is a single-seat fighter—on the hot, arid desert runway, a bit nervous but definitely excited, I waited to take off. Well trained and well equipped, I had in my control the best air-superiority fighter in the world. Loaded with three tanks of fuel and armed with a 20mm, six-barrel Gatling autocannon and eight missiles, I knew that Iraq's

Mikoyen-Gurevich–built interceptors, though inferior, still posed a threat.

Then it was time. Holding the brakes tightly, I ran my engines up to 80 percent and checked my engine instruments. After a sweeping look around the cockpit, I made eye contact with my flight lead next to me and gave him a nod, indicating I was ready for takeoff. Releasing his brakes, he took off down the runway like bolt of lightning, leaving a billowing residual cloud of dust hanging in the air over the runway. Then it was my turn. I released my brakes, pushed my throttles forward until they couldn't go any farther, and felt the "kick in the pants" from the afterburners lighting through all five stages. With my engines at full burner, I shot down the runway through my flight lead's residual dust cloud. The dashed white lines marking the center of the runway first blurred then fast became a solid white line. Pulling the plane's nose up, I rocketed skyward. I looked and watched the runway become very small very fast.

After rendezvousing with a tanker and doing a midair refueling, we received word of a pair of Iraqi MiG-25 fighter planes headed toward the No-Fly Zone. When my flight lead told us to turn our tapes on, my adrenaline really began to surge. (The F-15C has an 8mm tape to record its head-up display—critical during combat, it allows the pilot to chase or evade while monitoring flight data and radar—and there is no small real-world implication when the pilot turns on the tape.) Heading southbound toward the 33rd parallel after taking off from an airfield, the Iraqi MiGs were now skirting the No-Fly Zone about twenty-five miles to the north. Increasing speed and altitude, we began an intercept course. Once we'd gotten to about seventy-five miles from their position, however, the Iraqi pilots, in an exercise of unarguable wisdom, turned off and headed northeast.

After that first combat mission, I remained in-country until mid-March 2001, missing my son's first Christmas, as great a sacrifice as any. After returning to the States, the Air Force sent me to a Night Vision Goggle Instructor course in Phoenix in September. Waking up on 11 September, I turned on the television and, with shock and anger, witnessed with the rest of America, madmen deliberately flying the second of two airplanes into the World Trade Center. Since all commercial air travel immediately stopped, I was ordered to complete my course and then get back to my home base as soon as possible. When commercial air travel finally resumed, I was aboard one of the first airliners back in the skies.

With my squadron, tasked for Operation Noble Eagle, I flew security patrols over Atlanta and Washington, D.C., in the wake of the attacks. From that day forward, it was game day and we were ready twenty hours a day. When not flying, we'd sit alert in case a scramble order came down. No one complained, even though it meant sleeping in full flight gear—including boots and antigravity suit—only helmet and gloves at the ready. Monotonous and not a little uncomfortable, we were nonetheless honored to do it.

In spite of the tragedy (or perhaps because of it), I've experienced a level of pride being part of the U.S. military that I can only call climactic. I've come to truly understand service—giving of oneself for the good of nation and neighbor, expecting nothing in return. And though the Air Force changed my squadron's initial orders to Afghanistan, where I'd have welcomed serving, it ultimately did not matter. Wherever they need us, I, like the rest of the men and women serving the country in uniform, am more than willing to go.

•••

BIOGRAPHY: *Captain John "Jack" Antedomenico was born in 1971 in Bridgeport, Connecticut. Two days after graduating from the Air Force Academy in 1994, Antedomenico married his fiancée, Marcy. They are the proud and happy parents of a two-and-a-half-year-old boy. Since completing his flight training in 1999, Captain Antedomenico has participated in both Operation Southern Watch and Operation Noble Eagle. At this writing, Captain Antedomenico is the Chief of Wing Training at the 33d Operations Support Squadron, 33d Fighter Wing.*

Cold Warrior

By Commander Steven Corley, USNR (ret.)

as told to Milo James

I am forever grateful for and proud of my service in the U.S. Navy, where I spent eight years fighting the Cold War. Grateful because I developed skills and instincts there providing me with a superlative "competitive advantage" in the private sector. Proud because, despite the absence of open hostilities, I played a daily role in protecting America from the serious threat then posed by the Soviet Navy, in particular regarding its ballistic-missile submarines. As a Navy pilot in the P-3 community—the P-3 Orion is a turbo-prop, land-based aircraft with antisubmarine warfare and antisurface warfare capabilities —I dealt with that enemy every day, flying real-world missions on real-world targets all over the world.

In 1986, assigned to VP-26, Patrol Wing 5, Atlantic Fleet, out of NAS Brunswick in Brunswick, Maine, I flew a great many missions away from home. Being East Coast–based, our mission included providing continuous surveillance and intelligence gathering concerning Soviet naval capabilities in the Barents, Norwegian, and Mediterranean Seas and the Atlantic Ocean. Concerned especially with Soviet submarines along our eastern seaboard (they were well within launch range of major American inland cities), we also kept a sharp eye on the

Soviet subs posing a threat to our carrier battle groups in the Mediterranean. During my tenure in the Navy, the Soviet threat was especially dramatic; Soviet doctrine emphasized nuclear weaponry, and the USSR possessed the world's then-largest nuclear-powered ballistic-missile submarine force

Perhaps too simply put, when assets from the East Coast P-3 community worked a mission, it often proceeded something like this. After the Soviet Northern Fleet deployed a submarine into the Barents Sea out of Murmansk, we'd pick it up on SOSUS, our underwater, early-warning, sound-surveillance system. When the submarine drove through the GIUK Gap—a watery chokepoint between the North Atlantic and Norwegian Sea near Greenland, Iceland, and the United Kingdom—the Brits would get involved. Out of Iceland, we'd track it into the British area of responsibility, the Brits would pick it up and track it down to France, then the French (we had to let them play even though France was not a NATO member), tracking the submarine, would lose it. Starting from scratch, a P-3 squadron out of Lajes, Azores—about eight hundred miles off the coast of Portugal—would find it again and hand-off to our guys out of Rota, Spain, and they'd track it through the Strait of Gibraltar into the Mediterranean, finally passing the baton to our assets out of Sigonella, Sicily.

One mission I flew out of Lajes underscores the seriousness with which we Cold War warriors (on both sides) took our jobs. One rainy afternoon, VP-26 was tasked with finding a Soviet surface ship, part of a surface action group (SAG) out of Murmansk. The good guys had tracked the SAG but somewhere northwest of Lajes lost track of a Kirov class cruiser—then the largest and most heavily-armed cruiser in the world. So, taking off from Lajes Field with a crew of eleven, we left the small island of Terceira behind and headed out over the choppy, gray North Atlantic in search of the SAG.

Flying under the low, threatening clouds, we finally located the SAG in the far reaches of our patrol area. "We ought to turn back," I thought, knowing that if the "Death Star" (our nickname for the Kirov) were anywhere near, it would be out of our patrol area. As if confirming my thought, suddenly a little radar blip on the screen indicated something at the edge of our radar horizon. Deciding to go for it, I banked my airplane and flew in the direction indicated by the radar screen. After 125 miles, we found her. Doing her full speed, about 30 knots, this massive nuclear/steam-turbine-propulsion warship sported, instead of its normal fantail profile, an odd, twelve-foot-long "rooster tail"–looking thing.

Dropping the P-3's nose toward the choppy, gray water, I flew low and began making passes over her so we could gather PHOTINT (Photographic Intelligence) using our "eight-point rig," allowing us to take pictures from different angles. But every single time I passed low over the Kirov's fantail to get a good shot, the camera jammed, or we were not quite in position, or something else went wrong.

After having done four or five low passes over the 820-foot behemoth, it became obvious I had really pissed off her captain. Our Sensor Three (our nonacoustic sensor operator), dropping his headphones, turned toward the cockpit suddenly and yelled, "He's locked us up! He's locked us up!" The battle cruiser's AK-630s—six-barrel Gatling autocannons with fully automated tracking capability—had locked on to us. As I swooped low over ship and waves, the antiair defense system tracked us, its deadly accurate AK-630s spinning around on their turrets.

Still, I had to make another pass; it was critical we get some decent photos of the new fantail addition. Given the gravity with which the Soviet ship's captain was taking our aerial "trespass," though, that next five minutes was the longest of my life. Flying low again over the menacing Kirov, I concentrated, trying to coordinate with my other two pilots while concerned also about the danger posed by the ship's weapon—it can fire four thousand or five thousand rounds per minute of high-explosive fragmentation or fragmentation tracer rounds. I needed to get us the hell out of there; we were way too far from Lajes, in the middle of nowhere, no other place to go. While all these thoughts ran through my mind, fully cognizant of the utterly defense-less position we were in, I suddenly felt a strange "presence" behind me. Compelled, I turned from my instruments and, looking over my shoulder, saw my entire crew standing there, staring at me.

"Mister Corley," they said, "we think we need to go now."

I looked at them for a moment and blinked. "One more shot guys. We'll get it and then we'll go home."

I brought the P-3 around for one more low pass over the Kirov, its guns tracking us all the way. Finally getting a good picture, I pulled up, banked hard, and turned back toward Lajes.

The Cold War was a serious matter; winning it required committed, honorable people. My military skills and the mindset engendered by that struggle have translated exceptionally well to my personal and professional life. My "competitive advantage" noted above boils down to two things. Foremost, my military service solidified my sense of honor, the virtue of doing a good job and standing up for what is right, no matter the cost. I recognized the second, more pragmatic, benefit only after joining the civilian world. There (in this ex-Navy pilot's experience) are likewise too many decision-making-challenged individuals. But military life forces a person, whether as an NCO or officer, to take nebulous information and, with limited time, analyze it and make a good decision from it. In time, that becomes a part of who you are. Of all the benefits derived from serving America in the Navy, I am most grateful for the inculcation of honor and disciplined efficiency, and for the pride I have knowing I did well that which needed doing.

•••

BIOGRAPHY: *CDR Steven Corley, USNR (Ret.), was born in 1960 in Morganton, North Carolina. After graduating in 1982 from the U.S. Naval Academy, Corley served as an active duty Navy aviator for eight years. After leaving active duty, Corley received his law degree. He is a life member of both the Naval Academy Alumni Association and National Rifle Association. A father of three and grandfather of one, Corley lives in Morganton with his wife, Karen.*

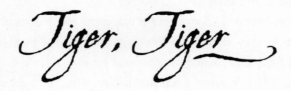

Tiger, Tiger

By "RUDY KIP"
as told to a friend

R udy sits at a coffee shop in a suburban area, where shopping malls dominate the landscape. He wants to tell his story—why he served and what he saw. Out on the patio of a java shop, the night sky illuminates with the beauty of the cosmos and Rudy begins:

"Tigers were there. Real jungle tigers. They weren't like the ones you see down at the zoo. These were wiry thin, grimy and raggedy looking. Tigers attuned to every whisper, light on their feet. This was the real thing, you know. In that jungle everything needed to be light on its feet. When 'in-country,' being wiry thin, light on your feet, and able to feast on a rodent meant living. Itwas survival."

Rudy, too, is wiry. He keeps a huge mug of coffee within his reach on a chilly night outside a coffee house. The mug he uses is his own, its once-ivory interior deeply stained, almost obsidian, from chronic use. It is over three decades since Rudy served in the U.S. Army, and he admits he never sleeps for long stretches even now, only in snatches —another legacy of his several tours of duty in the jungles of Southeast Asia.

"There was no special reason that I enlisted in the Army. I didn't know the difference. I didn't have a clue what the Army was. High

24

school was over and I was still at home. I figured that if I was going to have to take orders, I may as well get paid for it." He smiles a thin smile.

"I was ignorant of the ways of the world. I didn't have a clue at all. Politics wasn't my thing. I'd always been a pretty good athlete. No superstar, just pretty good. After the initial training the Army gave me, I volunteered for Special Forces."

Like the jungle tigers, Rudy was to prowl the tropical foliage of Southeast Asia. Quick on his feet, he was a natural for Special Forces. As Rudy tells it, Special Forces educated him.

"It wasn't formal education, you know, nothing like that. It was more like how to listen at night, how to see at night, and all the silent ways to do stuff. They taught us how to use various weapons and explosives and how to detect explosive booby traps, because the Vietcong, you know, they were damned masters of booby traps. The Vietcong could make booby traps out of anything. My Special Forces training lasted four months, though I did not know how to read or write until 1990."

He smiles another thin smile, a smile of gritty, quiet pride. Rudy's mastery of survival is rooted in his self-proclaimed illiteracy. He seems to share even more now with the jungle tigers. His survival there was instinctive, even primal.

Rudy explains that when he was discharged from the Army, he had no debriefing, no "deprogramming" or reeducation with respect to how to return to civilian (read: normal) life. Educated with four months of Special Forces training, he further perfected that education with twenty months of combat.

"Just like that, I was out-processed from Travis AFB. I was in one day, and the next day I was out on the streets of 'the world.' "

Rudy does not so much want to tell his stories, as he needs me to tell his stories. This, too, is the legacy of Vietnam. Rudy will spend the rest of his days deprogramming himself by sharing stories. It's how he survives in the concrete jungle here in "the world."

"'Skinned alive' is something more than an expression, you know. I saw it. I saw it up close, what it looks like for a human being to be skinned alive. You see that once, and you dread that torture more than anything else. Was I afraid? I was definitely afraid of being skinned alive. The body bags that we had were crap. They were really cheap stuff that tore really easily. It was dirty business picking up body parts, guts, and stuffing them in body bags that busted all the time. We scooped all sorts of junk into those body bags. Guess the government went with the lowest bidder to supply us our body bags. I wasn't afraid of much—but I did not want to be skinned alive."

To be eighteen, nineteen, twenty years old and have as one's foremost fear the very real possibility of being flayed? One might deal with the thought of scooping human intestines from the ground into a cheap body bag, but the notion of a human being enduring flaying? Rudy, a high school track-and-field enthusiast in 1968, one year later ranked being skinned alive as his number-one teenage fear. He learned to sleep in snatches while in-country. No wonder why. Surely it is better to stay awake than to dream. Continuing his deprogramming, Rudy tells what his young mind and body saw, did, withstood.

He swigs more coffee.

"We drank a lot of coffee during the day over there. Your mind wouldn't let you sleep deeply when you were in the jungles. We slept in snatches. You don't learn to do that; your mind does it for you. There were guys who liked to take guard duty. There were also some guys who you didn't want to take guard duty. You learn where to place your trust quickly, otherwise you're dead. The Army says I officially have seven kills. It is more likely well over twenty kills. You remember all the press that was given to the My Lai massacre? That stuff happened all the time. That poor fellow was just a scapegoat. There were orders we would get that would say, 'Hey, you guys go into these tunnels and don't use your weapons, don't use your flamethrower, and don't use your grenades, but take out the enemy.' The tunnels I am talking about were really complex, concrete-reinforced underground networks; no air-conditioning, but really sophisticated systems. Sometimes we'd get stupid orders like that. When it came down to it, we used everything we had, otherwise we'd have been mowed down. I don't fault anyone for stupid orders. Somewhere someone has to be responsible on paper. Using flamethrowers and grenades was ugly stuff down in the tunnels but not using them would have been more deadly. When you're in it, you do what you know you need to do to survive and we did. It was a mess; couldn't see and couldn't breathe down in those tunnels. We lost a lot of guys underground."

There is no bitterness. There is no rancor. Rudy doesn't offer a lot of judgment on what he saw. He states it all matter-of-factly. The body bags were cheap. He dealt with it. The government sent sleeping bags insulated for cold weather that they couldn't use. Solution: sleep under your poncho, propped up against a buddy. His boots were rarely dry, but the ponchos kept him relatively dry. Rudy doesn't punctuate his statements with gestures. He tells his story without passion, but neither does he do so prosaically. He was a teenager while in-country, and he did what he was trained to do. This man, who could neither read nor write, survived two tours in Vietnam.

His two R&R—rest and relaxation—trips, Rudy took to Taipei and Bangkok. He explains that he spent them getting drunk on cheap booze, remaining inexperienced about the ways of the world.

"When we were out on a mission we ate mostly C rations. That's some nasty stuff. We'd eat some Vietnamese food sometimes. I remember a lot of their foods being sweet. Their bread was really gritty. It was stone ground by hand and I think it was the stone particles that made it gritty."

Like his four-legged jungle counterpart, Rudy did not focus on feasting, but keeping light on his feet and alert. Light sustenance for the sake of fuel and coffee kept him going.

"You know I can't say that I didn't like being there. The drama, the excitement and adrenaline, all that trash. I was eighteen, nineteen, and twenty years old, and I did not know the politics and I didn't care. What did I know? When I got out of the Army in 1971 as an E-5, I was making $300 a month. You got $5 extra a month for overseas duty and an extra $15 a month for combat duty."

Finally, Rudy tells of his near miss at his nightmare:

"A group of nine of us went into Tay Ninh this one time searching for enemy activity. We were ambushed. To this day I could not tell you what happened to the other eight. That's the way things went over there. There I was captured. I was no value to them; a no-ranking regular Army guy like me was nothing. There was no way they were going to escort me across the country to North Vietnam to be their prisoner. We didn't take Vietcong prisoners, and they weren't going to keep me alive for long. My captors were sitting some distance away from me except for this one guy. I managed to get him in such a way that I broke his neck. I killed him. I tried to run. The next thing you know though, here come the rest of these guys. They caught me. They dislocated both of my shoulders and tied my arms behind my back at the elbows. I was in a lot of pretty unbelievable pain and unable to give any thought to escape anymore. 'OK, guys. Do what you have to do.' The next day I think—I lost track of time because of the pain—we were going along this really primitive trail, and we were ambushed by Special Forces guys. They weren't there to save me. They did not even know that I was there. I was damned lucky that I did not get shot up myself. I didn't have a shirt on and I was all covered in dirt; it was hard to tell which side I was on. Here I was on the ground as close as I could get and our guys were gunning my captors down. Who knows how I didn't get killed? This group of Special Forces guys called in a medevac for me. I was splinted up for about two months. A nineteen-year-old body has amazing recuperative capacity."

Of all the stories that Rudy has to tell, this is the most important to him. This is the one he needs to tell. By the length of a tiger's whisker and dumb chance he missed the fruition of his utmost fear of being skinned alive. Rudy never asked himself why he served in the Army or Vietnam. He was young and did what he was trained to do. He is proud of his combat duty and displays his Purple Heart combat status on his veteran's license plates. Doctors continue to dig shrapnel out of him every now and then. Like the wiry tigers in the wilds of Southeast Asia, he did what he had to do to survive. Now he paces our concrete jungle with the memories of what he survived.

•••

BIOGRAPHY: *"Rudy Kip" was born in and raised in the South. After graduating from high school in 1968, he enlisted in the U.S. Army. In January
1969, he was assigned to USARPAC in South Vietnam and then to the 25th
Infantry Division. Discharged in 1971, he was awarded two Purple Hearts,
an Army Commendation medal, and a Bronze Star for his service. A student
of martial arts, Kip now lives in a California city and is working on his
Master of Business Administration degree.*

That Others May Live

By Second Lieutenant Joseph Barnard, USAF

as told to Milo James

At about 0100 hours, I was flying aboard a U.S. Coast Guard C-130 transport plane five thousand feet above the Atlantic Ocean and six hundred miles east of the Bahamas. When the jump ramp in the aircraft's tail opened, the plane filled with cold, screaming air. Outside, the stars filled the night sky and the partial moon shone on the dark water below. The wind indicators we dropped—streamers with Chem-Lights so we could see them at night—showed little wind. My two team members and I jumped one after the other into the darkness, free-falling about eight seconds before pulling our ripcords. Our square canopies deployed, slowing us from a plummet to a smooth glide.

Below, the *Barbosi*, a seven-hundred-foot commercial freighter, sent a launch out to meet us, while the C-130 circled overhead. Steering ourselves toward the launch, whose crew could see the green and red Chem-Light lightsticks strapped to our bodies and our parachutes' silhouettes against the starry sky, we splashed into the water. The ocean was not choppy, but because hurricane Andrew was only three days away, the swells all around us were huge, as big as buildings; it was awesome! Ditching our parachutes, we swam with our medical gear to the launch and climbed its ladder.

Not long before we lifted off Homestead Air Force Base's runway twenty-five miles south of Miami, the *Barbosi*'s crew had radioed for help; their captain had taken ill and fallen unconscious, presumably with a heart problem. As we sped toward the *Barbosi*, we checked our gear, which included drugs, defibrillators, and other medical equipment we expected to need. Once aboard ship, we climbed eight decks to the bridge and found the captain in his nearby stateroom—all six-foot-seven, 420 pounds of him. The guy was huge! From the way he breathed, it was clear that his weight, complicated by onset diabetes, was the problem, not his heart after all.

While I worked the equipment and radio, communicating with our doctor aboard the circling C-130, Master Sergeant B., an Air Force reservist and Metro-Dade paramedic, our primary medic on this mission, went to work on the patient. We stabilized him as much as possible—we tried doing an insulin drop from the plane, but it missed the ship and we couldn't retrieve it—readying him for transport to a hospital in Nassau. First, though, we had to get the captain down from the tower. Eleven of us worked, sweating, for several hours, carrying his 420 deadweight pounds down eight flights of narrow, steep steps. By the time we reached the outside deck, it was morning and our own helicopters hovered over the ship.

Once we got the captain to an area of the ship where a helicopter could safely hover close enough to hoist him, we put him on the lowered hoist and they reeled him up. On the way back to shore, the captain actually "coded," his heart stopping, so we bagged him and intubated him with Lidocaine. When we finally reached the hospital in Nassau, about eighteen hours had passed since we received the call for help, but the fortunate captain lived.

We had spent the better part of twenty-four hours performing our respective tasks, without sleep, saving the *Barbosi*'s captain's life. Like any elite cadre of professionals, pararescue teams must do more than merely work well together; we have to know each other's thoughts, specialties, and training as we perform distinct tasks to create a single end result. The job is both awesome and moral. Working with guys willing to give up their own lives to save others creates a tremendous sense of job satisfaction. Because pararescue units are small, we have an especially high level of esprit de corps. From daily training and frequent "real world" operations, we grow to know one another closely.

The Air Force, which treats its people exceptionally well, further promotes job satisfaction, excellence, and camaraderie in general. It is amazing to me how well the Air Force values its people, in particular with respect to responsibility. We give our enlisted guys so much responsibility, both operationally and with respect to care of equipment and technology, and they are so well qualified to perform mission-critical functions that we'd literally fall apart without them.

On top of everything else, training for what we do is fun. While some people skydive, scuba, climb, or swim as an outside interest, we get to do all of that as part of our job. However fun the training, though, and however satisfying it is to save a life—be it an ill civilian, a lost hiker, or a soldier pinned down in combat—at the end of the day, it's a deadly serious job. Our mission takes us to the rescue of not only civilians, but also men and women on the battlefield. In fact, we lost an outstanding man, Jason Cunningham, a pararescueman from my own unit, during Operation Anaconda in Afghanistan, who did what any of the other men with whom I serve would do: put his own life at risk to save others. That's what pararescuemen do.

•••

BIOGRAPHY: *Born in 1964, Joseph Barnard served three years enlisted in the U.S. Army as an infantryman in the 82nd Airborne Division. Barnard served another ten years enlisted in the U.S. Air Force before being commissioned a second lieutenant. He is currently assigned to the 38th RQS, 347th Operations Group at Moody AFB, Georgia. Barnard is also currently working toward his Master's degree in Human Factors and Systems from Embry-Riddle University. He is husband to Megan and father to two boys.*

Fire in the Hole

By Lt. Col. Douglas Cameron (ret.)

The central coast of California in November and December has some of the most pleasant weather and beautiful scenery anywhere, and the day my story takes place was no exception. The low stratus clouds so typical of California's coastline had moved back out to sea at about the time my Titan II Combat Missile Crew and I reported for duty at 0730 this now bright and clear morning of November 30, 1967—leaving the rugged coastline visible for miles north and south of our temporary duty station of Vandenberg Air Force Base (AFB), just outside of Lompoc. Little did I know that my opportunities to enjoy these tranquil scenes were going to be limited for the next few days, especially today, because of one of the most harrowing and important events in my military career and in the history of the Titan II.

During the Cold War in 1967, the Titan II was America's biggest and most powerful ICBM (Intercontinental Ballistic Missile)— 102 feet high, 430,000 pounds of thrust, capable of reaching any target on earth.

Our missile had been selected at random by the Strategic Air Command (SAC) as part of a program to confirm the operational readiness of missiles and crews. Three crews were selected by competition from the site that normally staffs the missile selected. My crew and I, and the two other crews selected, were from the 374th Strategic Missile Squadron at Little Rock, Arkansas. The selected missile was pulled from its home silo and sent to Vandenberg AFB where it was placed in an operational silo and readied for alert status—but with a dummy warhead. The three crews cycle through their normal duty schedule for at least two weeks, awaiting a call to launch.

It was my crew's turn in the duty cycle on November 30, 1967. We reported for work as usual, and as any Combat Missile Crew does, we waited. Except that waiting in the military while on duty always means some form of busywork—clean this, polish that, inspect something.

We were well into our busywork at about 1000 (10:00 a.m.) when the loud speakers broke the tedium with our call-sign, which meant that the message was for our missile only. (If it was a fleetwide message, it would have been SAC's call-sign, which at the time was Sky King.) I don't remember our exact call-sign at the time because they changed daily for security reasons, but it was probably something like Bright 21 (two-one). So the speakers blared, "Bright 21, Bright 21, standby to copy [encoded] message." (The formats and codes changed frequently also.) A code was transmitted that we had to decode within one minute—no more. If it was to be a launch, that code would authorize us to take the keys from around our (mine and Lt. James Swayze's) necks, place them in the launch panel, and turn them simultaneously to launch the missile. This time, that launch code was transmitted, and we—Lt. Swayze, Deputy Combat Missile Crew Commander; SSgt. Lyle Groth, the Ballistic Missile Analysis Technician (BMAT); TSgt. Robert Turner, the Missile Facilities Technician; and I—all went to work as the well-trained crew that we were. Sgts. Turner and Groth had both been through this before. However, there were problems downrange—somewhere in the four thousand miles between Vandenberg AFB and the Kwajalein Islands, the target, there was something that the Air Force didn't want to sink with a ten thousand–pound cement warhead, maybe even a Soviet trawler. So we had a hold placed on our launch—highly unusual for a ballistic missile crew just told to launch its missile. Eventually we were told that we could launch at 1300 hours (1:00 p.m.).

At 1300, we went through the checklist again, Lt. Swayze and I turned the keys and released them, and we began watching the sequence of lights start moving across the board, which would in about one minute result in the lighting of the "Fire Engine" light and the departure of the missile. We watched almost casually as the sequence progressed, because we had been through this dozens of times in the simulator. That training, however, is worthless if it does not prepare you for all foreseeable emergencies; but when the sequence arrived at the "Thrust Mount Soft" light, the unforeseeable did happen. There was no "Thrust Mount Soft" light or "Fire Engine" light—though I did have a "Fire in Launch Duct" light and an "Engine Fire" light, followed closely by myriad other red and yellow lights and a loud, god-awful klaxon—*BUZZ! GONG! BUZZ! GONG!* I kept trying to shut it off (it was very distracting), but it kept coming back on—with more flashing and twinkling lights. Flash! Flash!

I called out, "Fire in engine!" and "Fire in launch duct!" but Col. Pickle in the Command Post thought I said "Fire Engine," which would have meant that launch was imminent, and he, therefore, told CINCSAC (the commander in chief of SAC) to "standby for launch." I didn't have time to correct him. *BUZZ! GONG! BUZZ! GONG!* Flash! Flash!

Even with all the ruckus going on, we still had absolutely no indication that the missile had departed, or even if it was still in the silo. The launching system was so automatic that it was assumed that it would run its course, the "Fire Engine" light would come on, the rocket engine would go to its full 430,000 pounds of thrust, within six seconds the explosive bolts securing the missile to the earth would let go, and the missile would just fly noisily away.

Meanwhile, we were still at *BUZZ! GONG! BUZZ! GONG!* Flash! Flash! Then came the "Abort" light, which meant that the circuitry connecting the missile to the silo was still there, the missile had been at full power for at least six seconds, and MAY have still been at full power, but was still attached to Mother Earth. Were the silo doors still open or closed? Was the second stage about to ignite, possibly in a closed silo? Were we about to be evaporated by a rocket at its full 430,000 pounds of thrust and an almost-full load of fuel? Would the blast doors hold? SSgt. Lyle Groth, the BMAT, had to run over to another room across the hall to confirm whether or not the missile was still in the silo, which he did, and it was—costing us several seconds. (He wouldn't have had to run and check at our base in Arkansas, because he would have had the information at his panel—Vandenberg had an older setup.) I then told Lt. Swayze to start the Abort Checklist. We were still BUZZING, GONGING, and FLASHING, but we completed the checklist twenty-four seconds after the "Abort" light—the final step of which is to push the shut-down button, which turns off the fuel valves and closes the silo doors.

My next thought was, Was that missile about ready to fly?—with the silo doors closed? I pushed the button, lights started to go out, the klaxon finally stopped, and we got to the business of "safeing" the silo, making sure nothing more was burning or in danger of exploding.

The chaos didn't end there though. SAC, the Command Post, and probably the cashier at the BX (Base Exchange) were asking where the missile was. In the silo? Mach two downrange? Situated on top of the silo? Nobody, but apparently us, knew. A general at an observation post a mile away said he saw the doors open, the doors close, and lots of fire, but he didn't see the missile. A major with him said, "You missed it, sir!" The fire department personnel assigned to cover the launch saw so much fire they ran off like scared dogs until ordered at gunpoint by a colonel at Range Control to go back and see if the crew in the silo needed any help—or rescue.

They finally agreed with us that the missile was still in the silo, after someone got up the courage to look down the hole. Meanwhile, we sat in toxic fumes for seven hours until released, but were then sequestered for three days during the investigation that ensued. The Air Force, the engineers, the contractors, and the BX cashier were all thoroughly confused and dismayed. This had never happened before, and I was accused of all kinds of malfeasance.

Six months later, though, I was absolved of any wrongdoing because they found a problem in the solid state circuitry of the timer systems that should have sent the "explode" message to the explosive bolts but did not. My crew and I had done our job, and done it well, even in the face of the unforeseeable. The malfunction was found to be virtually fleetwide.

I was later asked, if called to do that job again, would I, considering how I had been treated by the Air Force. My reply was a resounding, "Yes!" The Air Force was just doing its job. It had to make sure that its missiles and its crews were unconditionally ready, and that we had the resolve and the capacity to act when called upon. Those operational tests, and how the Air Force responded to the quality or success of those tests, were an important part of telling the world that we were ready.

••

BIOGRAPHY: *Douglas Cameron, Sr., was born in Green Lake, Washington, on January 5, 1934. He enlisted in the U.S. Air Force on December 3, 1952. Cameron's career spanned thirty-one years, in which he rose in rank to lieutenant colonel. His duty stations spanned the globe, including Germany and Vietnam. In full retirement now, he lives with his wife of forty-six years, Joan, in Orangevale, California, where he enjoys building radio-controlled airplanes, fishing, gardening, and spending time with his three grown sons, Michael, Bruce, and Douglas, Jr.*

The Point of Go-No-Go

By James Elmer

as told to Anthony Elmer

As a pilot in the Strategic Air Command (SAC), my job was to pilot a flying gas tank. The official Air Force name is the KC-135 Stratotanker. SAC has a lot of rules and regulations when it comes to flying, especially concerning in-flight, aerial refueling. SAC has a procedure for everything and numerous checklists to complete for its operations. There is no room for independent thought when you fly in the military—you must go by "the book."

Late August 1982, my crew finally got some rest at Hickam AFB (Air Force Base), Hawaii. We had been on various refueling missions in the Pacific, supporting B-52 Bombers in Guam, and we were on our way home to Mather AFB in Sacramento. We got up before dawn and were at base operations where we received our orders. We were to upload our aircraft with 20,000 gallons of fuel and rendezvous with a C-5A Galaxy 1,000 miles east of Hawaii and offload 12,000 gallons. The KC-135 weighs 130,000 pounds before fuel and cargo. The 20,000 gallons of fuel weighs 140,000 pounds. It's easy to do the math; the fuel we were carrying weighed more than we did. That is not so bad, except we did not have water for a water-injected takeoff. The KC-135 is not equipped with the fan engines its civilian counterparts have; we rely on injecting 2,000 pounds of water into each of the airplane's four engines to increase thrust for takeoff. Hickam did not have the purified water, so my copilot and navigator reviewed the charts and decided to take off with the heavy load. I reviewed the aircraft performance charts and weather information and agonized over the data because it was scheduled to be eighty-two degrees for takeoff, and we had little margin for error. (The warmer the temperature, the less dense the air. The less dense the air, the lower the performance of the aircraft engines and the ability of the wings to generate lift.)

The preflight check went fine. Fuel loaded and weight and balance completed, we were ready for taxi, and my copilot received clearance for takeoff. Before we got out of the chocks, base operations called us to hold for passengers. We can take up to twenty passengers if we have seats. I told operations we were heavy on fuel, and we couldn't really take any more weight. Operations informed me that another plane had maintenance problems and these passengers were high priority. Eight senior Air Force officers and their families got on board. We allotted two hundred pounds per person, including luggage, increasing our gross weight by four thousand pounds, but they had lots of luggage. I began to sweat this flight—especially considering that the lives of the families seated on this plane were my responsibility.

Nevertheless, the airplane felt good. The sky was clear, and we were going home. The performance manuals said we could take off, but again we had not counted on the extra weight of twenty passengers. The extra weight nagged at me, and while we were holding before takeoff, I reviewed the performance charts again. My copilot told me, "The book says we can do it." Every pilot knows his "air sense," his intuition about each flight, overrides "the book."

Though my "air sense" was screaming that something was going to go wrong, tower cleared us for takeoff and gave us the wind direction and speed and noted a perfect temperature of eighty-two degrees Fahrenheit. We took the runway and I pushed the throttles up and scanned the instruments: RPM, fuel flow, exhaust gas temperature. The copilot's duties include monitoring the instruments and the "go-no-go point," a fixed distance down the runway at which an airplane, on reaching a certain minimum speed, can either take off or abort safely with the remaining available runway.

After we reached the "go-no-go point," an unusual and ominous thing happened. The airplane seemed to act sluggish. The airspeed indicator barely moved. I tapped the glass cover, thinking it was stuck. The copilot pushed the throttles to the full position. Still the airspeed failed to noticeably increase. We couldn't abort, because at the end of the runway at Hickam is a twenty-foot drop into the Pacific Ocean. An abort would mean certain death for us. I looked down at the airspeed indicator, my pulse rapidly increasing. The airspeed indicator read 118 knots. We needed 121 to rotate, and the overrun was coming into my windscreen. I quickly told the copilot I was extending my takeoff into the overrun. We had no choice. The overrun is paved surface, not constructed to support the weight of the aircraft, and used for emergencies only. Extending takeoff into the overrun, however, meant that we'd literally risk running the plane over the cliff. I continued the takeoff into the overrun and flew the airplane ten to fifteen feet off the water for at least half a mile before I got enough airspeed to rotate.

When we cleared the runway/overrun, I instructed the copilot not to raise the gear, because the extra drag from the gear doors opening would make our situation worse. The cockpit was extremely tense and I screened out all distractions. Our carefully rehearsed procedures were abandoned. I told my copilot to leave the flaps alone until we were safe, because we needed all the lift we could get. If we couldn't attain the lift, we'd be crashing in the water. Flying so close to the water with gear down kept us in "ground effect"—meaning the effect of the water's surface on the aircraft's wings increases the plane's aerodynamics—and luckily we climbed to altitude without further problems.

But imagine the commotion created by that half mile we needed over the bay at only ten to fifteen feet above the water in order to attain the lift. Though we may have been internally panicking in the cockpit, boats, surfers, sun worshippers, and wading tourists furiously scrambled to get out of our way! Who in their position wouldn't have? This huge aircraft looked like it was going to clip or crash into you as it seemed to head for an impact in the waves.

On climb-out, one of the passengers, a colonel, came up to the cockpit and told me he was going to report me to the wing commander and have me taken off flying status for that dangerous stunt.

When we finally arrived at Mather AFB, in California, we were met by the staff duty officer and the group operations officer. They told me that there were numerous reports of our low-flying airplane, a serious violation. In addition, Hickam and Honolulu Airport had filed air restriction violations. True to his word, the colonel had filed a complaint in person and asked for a complete investigation.

Next day, the squadron commander and the group commander informally took me off flying status until they conducted a complete investigation. They informed me that, as an aircraft commander, I should never have extended my takeoff into the overrun, and certainly never flown the airplane over the water with the gear down. Over the next few weeks, the investigators reviewed our fuel logs, maintenance records, interviewed the crew, checked all engines and instruments, and reviewed all the information from the flight data recorder, and forwarded all applicable data to Boeing for analysis.

A few weeks later I stopped by the squadron to check my crew box. There were the usual updates for the manuals and safety tips. Somewhere buried in the paperwork was a typed message from Boeing Flight Test, which ended with this sentence: "After reviewing the information you provided, it is our opinion that the exemplary flying skills of Major Elmer probably averted a major aircraft incident."

* * *

BIOGRAPHY: *James Elmer was born in 1945 in Iowa. First a navigator in the Iowa National Guard, Elmer later transferred to the Air Force Reserves, flying missions around the globe. Now a lawyer, Elmer retired from the Air Force Reserves in 1987 with over two thousand hours' flight time. He resides in Sacramento, California, with his wife, Kris, and their three children.*

A Sailor Remembers the "Mindanao"

—By Captain Carlo Anthony Delaurentis, USN (ret.)—

as told to Milo James

10 November 1944, 0800 hours. The hot sun overhead beat down as I pulled away from my ship, the USS *Mindanao* (ARG-3) piloting a liberty launch on the eight o'clock run to the beach. The *Mindanao*, a repair ship operating in the South Pacific supporting naval forces in the fight against Japan, was anchored in Seeadler Harbor, Manus, Admiralty Islands, northeast of New Guinea. Amidst a harbor filled with about two hundred other ships, anchored about 350 yards to our ship's portside was the USS *Mount Hood* (AE-11), a nearly 460-foot Wrangell-class munitions ship. A floating ammunition depot, she carried about thirty-eight hundred tons of ammunition, including bombs, powder, various projectiles, depth bombs, and fuzes.

Not originally scheduled to make this particular run, ferrying our postal clerk and supply clerk ashore to pick up mail and supplies, I told the coxswain of a launch similar to mine that I'd take the eight o'clock run since something was wrong with his boat. Shortly before 0900, while I waited in the launch for the mail clerk and supply clerk to complete their business ashore, a tremendous explosion resounded in the harbor behind me. Whirling around, I saw a humongous orange and yellow fireball emanating from where the USS *Mount Hood* had been anchored. A black-and-gray mushroom cloud of smoke billowed outward about one hundred feet and rose into the sky seven thousand feet totally obscuring the immediate area. Over the water, smoky trajectories shot through the air, marking the course taken by twisted chunks of ship, shrapnel, and blown munitions before splashing into the water hundreds of yards away or thudding into the decks of other ships and injuring and killing men.

The *Mount Hood*, blown to smithereens, literally disappeared. The only significant remnant—as I understood it—besides the telltale oil slick floating on the harbor's surface, was a section of the *Mount Hood*'s hull in a trench in the bottom of the harbor, the muddy intaglio eerily reminiscent of the ship's position before the explosion. Flying projectiles from the destroyed craft blasted the portside hull of the *Mindanao*, which would certainly have capsized had it not been for seven minesweepers moored to her starboard side, and damaged dozens of other ships in the harbor.

Immediately pulling away from the beach, I sped back to my ship. As I approached her, joining several dozen other small craft carving their way through the oil slick to assist, the *Mindanao*'s damage became clear. Dozens of holes, large and small, pockmarked her hull and superstructure. It looked like she had been used for artillery practice. My fortune did not escape me; had I not taken the eight o'clock run to the beach, I might have been among the wounded or dead. In fact, the men whom I'd relieved, those originally scheduled to take the morning run to shore, all died in the explosion.

On deck, it was chaos, men rushing about treating the wounded; bagging bodies; and fishing men, alive and dead, out of the water. Back aboard ship, I pitched in. One guy we fished out of the water did not have his shoes. When we went to the spot on deck where he'd been working on a small boat at the time of the explosion, we found the shoes still on deck, right where he'd been standing; he'd literally been blown out of his shoes! When, finally, after hours of work by hundreds of men, things calmed down, I sat down. I had lost several friends in the explosion, and took the time to write their mothers to tell them that their sons received a proper burial.

Earlier that year, I had submitted an application for acceptance into the Navy's dental program at Northwestern University. That afternoon, when we finally had the chance to tend to more mundane matters, I learned my application had been accepted. Because my orders were to report to Northwestern on I January, I left the *Mindanao* a few days later and, traveling eastward around the globe, arrived in San Francisco in December. Before reporting to Northwestern, I took a train across the country to Pennsylvania to spend a few weeks with my family and visit nearby families of shipmates who'd died, whom I was unable to write earlier, to tell them their sons received proper burials.

The still-lucid memory of that day remains with me today, at the age of eighty-five, and now and then I think about the friends I lost, and pray for them. It was absolutely tragic, and so far as I know, there are still conflicting accounts to explain the explosion. Regardless of the cause, though, many good men died that day serving their fellow sailors and country, the sobering price of freedom.

•••

BIOGRAPHY: *Carlo Anthony Delaurentis, D.D.S., was born in Wayne, Pennsylvania, in 1917. In 1942, Carlo enlisted in the U.S. Navy. During his enlistment, the Navy accepted Carlo into its dental program at Northwestern University in Chicago, where he met a Yeoman Third Class named Margaret, whom he married. After more than thirty years, Carlo retired from the Navy at the rank of captain. Carlo enjoys his time with his wife of fifty-six years and his six sons, nine grandchildren, and two great-grandchildren, in Coronado, California.*

Field Ingenuity

By "Ted"

as told to Milo James

In December 1966, I was medical supply officer at ASCOM (Army Support Command) Depot in northwestern South Korea, midway between Seoul and Inch'on. One Saturday afternoon, while on duty as officer of the day, I took a call from the Office of the Surgeon General, EUSAK (Eighth U.S. Army, Korea) in Seoul. A diphtheria outbreak had hit the capital and its surrounding areas, and the EUSAK Surgeon General's office wanted antidiphtheritic to combat the highly contagious, life-threatening disease. I immediately contacted our storage officer and reported back to the EUSAK Surgeon General's office how much of the medicine we had. Saying that it wasn't even close to sufficient, the colonel told me what he needed. "Fine sir, we'll get it," I assured him. I called the Defense Personnel Support Center (DPSC) in Philadelphia, which had logistical responsibility for ordering and storing medical supplies for all the armed forces worldwide, and double ordered, just in case of any snafus. Having located the medical depot nearest us with the medication, DPSC cut a requisition for a shipment to our location.

Giving no second thought to the relatively uncomplicated, albeit urgent, order, I went down to the officers' club for dinner. I'd heard the

O-Club received a shipment of especially good beef—a rare commodity in Korea then—and had been anticipating a good steak all afternoon. Just as I cut into my steak, the waiter approached, saying I had a phone call at the bar. Slightly annoyed, I went to the bar and picked up the phone. A southern accent on the other end identified the speaker as Air Force Major So-And-So in Okinawa. "Captain," he said, "I've got a request from Philadelphia to get some antidiphtheritic up to you boys just as fast as I can. Will you authorize a jet fighter to carry that?"

Initially taken aback—majors typically do not ask captains to authorize anything—I thought, "What the hell? This is an emergency and the colonel told me to get it here ASAP." Possibly violating both Army and Air Force regulations, I said, "Major, I do authorize your use of a jet fighter to fly in that medicine. Give me your flight information so we can coordinate this with the receiving facility in Japan." Taking the information, I called Japan, then the Surgeon General's office, and then returned to my steak, thinking only of the need to apprise the EUSAK Surgeon General's office that the medicine would arrive Monday at Osan Air Base (about thirty miles south of Seoul) via the "milk run"—the troops' moniker for the daily supply and mail flight from Japan.

Because of Korea's rugged terrain, nascent infrastructure—in 1966 there were few decently paved roads—and the timeliness of the mission, it seemed more expeditious to take a helicopter to Osan instead of a jeep. (That I enjoyed flying in helicopters had nothing to do with my decision, of course.) Monday morning, I called the nearby medevac detachment, which had several helicopters, and explained the situation to the officer in charge, another major. Though, for whatever reason, he had a serious case of the ass and gave me a lot of grief at first, not wanting his choppers used, he finally—after I threw around the weight of the EUSAK Surgeon General's office—complied and assigned a pilot to take me and my staff sergeant to Osan.

We arrived at Osan AB about the same time as the milk run. After all other cargo had been off-loaded, the Air Force technical sergeant in charge of the off-load told us our medicine was not aboard. Climbing into the DC-3's cargo area, I looked around to confirm, jumped down from the plane, and walked to a generic-government-looking airfield office.

First, I called Japan and asked them to check out where we'd arranged to have the medicine stored. It was there. Very politely, I told them the problem they had caused, and they assured me it would be on tomorrow's plane. Then I called Seoul. Reaching the colonel—a "full bird"—in the Eighth Army Surgeon General's office with whom I had been communicating all along, I matter-of-factly explained what happened. "We've got a little problem here, sir. For some reason the medicine did not get on the milk run. It's still in Japan and will be delivered here tomorrow."

"No, Captain, we don't have a little problem," he rejoined. "YOU have a big problem."

"What do you mean, sir?"

"Well," he began with the tone of a full-bird colonel who did not get what he wanted, "the EUSAK Surgeon General has already told the mayor of Seoul, AND the Korean media, AND the *Stars and Stripes*"—the venerable, privately owned, armed forces–focused newspaper—"that the medication is on its way and they're all expecting the stuff to be delivered. Today!"

I asked him what he wanted me to do about that, and he said, "Captain, that's YOUR problem," and hung up.

Sweating bullets (not easy to do in December in Korea), I got off the phone and back on the helicopter with my staff sergeant. As we lifted off the helipad heading to Seoul with only the medicine we brought from our depot, my staff sergeant asked, "Sir, what the hell are you gonna do?"

"Doesn't antidiphtheritic require a quality-control check before it's shipped to medical units for use?" I replied.

"Well, yeah. It does, as a matter of fact, sir."

"We could tell them that's what we're doing," I began. "But, we don't have testing capability at the depot."

"Well," he offered thoughtfully, grinning, "we know that, but they don't."

Deciding that was the only plausible course of action, I sat back in the helicopter, watching the barren Osan lowlands give way to the rugged Kwangju mountains as we neared Seoul. After touching down, I opened the helicopter door. The sergeant and I stepped out into the chilly air. An unexpected roar of applause from a cheering mob and a military band—striking up some John Philip Sousa anthem—shocked the hell out of us. Korean and *Stars and Stripes* reporters snapped pictures, camera bulbs flashing all over the place, and journalists jockeyed for positions in front of the crowd to levy their prepared questions. It sounded like halftime at a football game. We met the mayor of Seoul, who, standing with the EUSAK Surgeon General, gripped our hands and pumped them gratefully, smiling. I handed our single box of medicine to the EUSAK Surgeon General, who then presented it to the mayor.

One reporter, however, an ensign from *Stars and Stripes*, pressed us, a curious expression on his face. Seeing the single box we off-loaded from the helicopter, he asked, "Is that all?" I told him no, there was more to come. But he continued, "How come it's not here?" The time for "Truth or Dare" had come. I stood taller, stuck out my chest, jutted out my jaw, got in the ensign's face, and said, "Ensign, what is it you do not understand about quality control? If we issue medicine that is in any way defective, it can hurt people, not help them. I'll tell you one last time, the remainder of the shipment will be disbursed as soon as the quality control check is completed."

Turning, I walked into an office with my staff sergeant, but the ensign was damned persistent. Following us in, he began his line of questioning again. "This guy is like a bloodhound and could cause a major problem," I thought. The only way to get rid of him was to get the hell out of there, so I told him—this time less threateningly since that obviously had no effect the first time—"Ensign, we would love to stay and talk to you, but we have to leave now. Our pilot has informed us that he needs to get our asses back on that chopper because there's some kind of medical emergency and medevac needs their chopper back immediately."

The sergeant and I paid our obligatory respects to the colonel. "Captain," he said, "call me immediately when you get back." The ensign either did not think to ask why they could not use another chopper or he finally wised up when he overheard the colonel's tone of voice. For whatever reason, he kept his mouth shut. Next day, of course, the medicine came on the milk run, and I sent someone to pick it up and take it to Seoul.

My reason for that bit of inveiglement was, since the antidiphtheritic was to arrive next day—already having been quality checked, of course—no harm would follow, and if he'd reported what had happened, it could only unnecessarily embarrass the EUSAK Surgeon General's office as well as the EUSAK Surgeon General. I saw no point in that, either altruistically or self-interestedly (it would not have been exactly the best career move). The problem, of course, could have been avoided from the beginning had the good intentions behind locating and distributing the medication to the Korean civilians not been politicized. But, what the hell? Korea was a boring place for GIs in those days, so while saving who-knows-how-many lives, we had ourselves a little adventure and a bit of fun, not to mention getting to fly around in a helicopter. Thanks, Sergeant F.

•••

BIOGRAPHY: *"Ted" was born in 1940 and raised in western Pennsylvania. After resigning his commission in the Army, Ted pursued a career in business. Ted and his wife of forty years have two daughters, a son, and five (soon to be seven) grandchildren. A fighter and courageous man, Ted recently made a miraculous and complete recovery from a bout with what he was told was incurable cancer.*

Marine Corps Meets Peace Corps

— By Gunnery Sergeant Frank Buday, USMC —

(ret.)

The U.S. military has a well-deserved reputation as one of the best-trained, best-disciplined, and best-equipped armies in the world. Since the Revolution, it has fought valiantly to protect this country, maintaining its oath of fealty to defend and protect the Constitution. The courage and honor of the American soldier, sailor, airman, or Marine is a constant. Yet, there exist aspects of the military of which the average citizen is unaware. Not only do members of the military go to war to protect our freedom, but they also perform unknown, rarely heralded humanitarian missions, which, if acknowledged, are often only a sound bite on the evening news. These operations protect and help Americans in foreign lands and provide health and comfort to citizens of other nations.

Part of the 26th Marine Expeditionary Unit (26 MEU), I left Camp Lejeune just before Thanksgiving 1996. After a ten-day Atlantic crossing, we reached the U.S. Naval Station at Rota, Spain, for reprovisioning and entry into the Mediterranean. Passing through the Pillars of Hercules, we zigzagged to our first port, Trieste, Italy, for Christmas liberty. As one of two senior enlisted Marines in the Joint Intelligence Center aboard 26 MEU's command ship, the USS *Nassau*

(LHA-4), I was in charge of the day shift. Working from 0430 to 1700, we read, studied, analyzed, condensed, and prepared message traffic received the night before for an 0800 intelligence brief for our commander and his staff each morning. My duties also included ensuring my people remained cognizant of their duties and fully knowledgeable regarding our area of responsibility—all Adriatic countries south to Turkey. Though we did not study the northern European countries in depth—no one thought we might have to invade and conquer Switzerland or France, after all—we kept an eye on them vis-à-vis their interests in North African, Middle Eastern, and Adriatic countries.

While our mission in the Adriatic was to provide "a forward deployed military response to situations that may occur in Bosnia, Croatia, and Serbia that may have an impact upon the European Union and NATO," former Yugoslavian republics were relatively quiet and calm, initially. By mid-January, however, having predicted Kosovo and Macedonia were ready to explode, we kept a sharp eye on them. Albania didn't "feel" right either and raised hairs on our necks. We began collecting historical data, current events, and news about the political situation in Albania and constructed relational line and block charts of all in-country governmental and political agencies.

On March 3, 1997, rioting broke out in Tirane, Albania's capital. President Sali Berisha's government went into hiding, law and order disappeared, and looters broke into armories throughout the country. 26 MEU was called in to effect Operation Silver Wake, a Non-Combatant Evacuation Operation (NEO), to evacuate U.S. citizens and provide security-force protection to the U.S. embassy in Tirane.

In the hierarchy of evacuations, U.S. citizens *always* have priority, followed by allied countries' citizens, third nations' citizens, non-aligned countries' citizens, and, finally, hostile countries' citizens. For the next two weeks, we evacuated approximately twenty-seven hundred people comprising over twenty-five nationalities, including Americans, French, British, Italians, Swiss, Russians, Romanians, Bulgarians, Turks, Greeks, Iranians, Iraqis, and Pakistanis. Most evacuees came through the USS *Nassau*, though the other two ships in our Amphibious Readiness Group, the USS *Nashville* (LPD-13) and the USS *Pensacola* (LSD-38), also processed their share. In processing evacuees for transport to Italy, we screened them and collected as much information as possible regarding the situation in-country, obtaining snapshots of information concerning the operation.

On the second day alone, we processed over 375 U.S. citizens, mostly embassy, USAID, and Peace Corps personnel. The Peace Corps volunteers were my favorite. One couple I processed, in their late thirties or early forties and quite nice, I was able to sit with and have a very pleasant talk with them. Later that evening, I saw them leaving the ship, on their way to Italy. As they passed me and I again said thank you, good luck, and good-bye, the woman performed *namaste* (the Sanskrit word means, roughly, "I bow in humble honor to the Light within you")—a gesture of kindness or gratitude performed by pressing one's palms together before the heart and slightly bowing the head—which surprised me. Though I recognized it, I did not return the gesture as I should have, and I will always carry a feeling of disappointment for not returning that beautiful gesture.

By mid-March, the political situation in Zaire, Africa, had also deteriorated and 26 MEU was asked to provide the same NEO services in the west-coast African country. Being Marines, we'd torn from our dictionary the page containing the word "no," and 26 MEU headed for Zaire, leaving a "B" command—a splinter detachment created from the main command group—and one ship, the *Nashville,* off the coast of Albania. As a "B" command member, I had forty-five minutes after the orders came down to pack everything I'd need for the next few months—clothes, books, computer, printer, reference materials, and all supplies. Grabbing my weapons from the armory, I locked and secured everything I was leaving behind and said good-bye to my comfort zone.

The intel shop in "B" command consisted of five people: Captain T., an excellent officer; Lance Corporal A., a pretty good kid who had his own subscription to the *New York Times Book Review;* Staff Sergeant P.

and Staff Sergeant S., both Interrogator-Translators (ITTs); and me. The two ITT staff sergeants rounded out my HUMINT (Human Intelligence) Exploitation team (HET). Like everyone else in the "B" command, I wore many different hats: I functioned as intelligence chief, sole counterintelligence representative, and senior HET representative; I provided intelligence briefs every morning; and I performed any other job requiring intelligence support. The best thing, though, was my new work hours: no more 0430 to 1700 every day of the week. This time I worked 1800 to 0600.

Remaining aboard the *Nashville* more than two months, I sailed in squares doing "ModLocs"—Miscellaneous Operational Details, Local Operations—off the coast of Albania, while Staff Sergeants P. and S. stayed ashore, liaising between the embassy staff and the Marines and analyzing, identifying, and locating incoming points of fire—*sniping* is not an accurate term in this case, since the Albanians were less-than-adequate marksmen—from Albanians outside the embassy wire.

By late April, the situation had calmed down, all intel people were aboard ship, and we lapsed into a routine; the only excitement was a visit from Congressman Sonny Bono of California (which I missed since he came during the day when I was sleeping). "B" command having finally been relieved in May of all duties in Albania pertaining to Operation Silver Wake and having refitted for our cruise home, we soon passed through the Pillars of Hercules again, about 0500 hours. Standing on deck, I watched Gibraltar pass by on the starboard side and the mountains of Africa far off to port.

Though out of the Mediterranean and crossing the Atlantic, we still provided intel briefs and monitored the situation in Albania. I continued to work my now-routine hours and found a way to make that night shift work for me. Forward of the intel center was the command briefing room and beyond that the captain's bridge on the third deck, which, of course, faced the ship's bow, providing an unobstructed view of the ocean. The glassed-in bridge measured about eight feet by twenty-five feet and sported a large, comfortable captain's chair—resembling a luxurious, adjustable, comfortable barber's chair —bolted to the deck.

The moon was three days shy of full, and every night from 0100 to 0230 I'd go to the bridge, kick back in the captain's chair, and watch the moonlight play off the ocean before me as we steamed forward along the watery moonlit path before us. The lunar reflections, glimmering and bouncing, breaking into a million sparkling gems, mesmerized and relaxed me. I found the beauty so meaningful, so indescribable, that I asked myself over and again whether the months aboard ship were a fair exchange for those couple of hours each night, whether it is worth it to exchange an irreplaceable part of one's life for beauty. After nine days crossing the Atlantic like that, the answer was unequivocal: absolutely.

•••

BIOGRAPHY: *Frank Buday, born in 1951, was raised in Youngstown, Ohio. Influenced by the Leon Uris novel* Battle Cry, *he enlisted in the Marine Corps in 1969. He married his wife, Deborah, in 1977. After more than twenty-one years as a Marine, Buday retired at the rank of Gunnery Sergeant in the field of counterintelligence. He attended Campbell University and received a BA in History in June 2001.*

First Rescue

By Staff Sergeant (P) Scott Carmack, USAF

as told to Milo James

When I joined the Air Force, I initially intended to become an air-traffic controller. But when, during basic training, I had the opportunity to get out of an afternoon of basic training to test for Air Force Pararescue, everything changed and my fate was sealed. Since PJs—parajumpers, members of an Air Force Pararescue team—conduct conventional and unconventional operations under all possible conditions, the training is long and intense. After basic training, I completed a series of "high-speed" courses, called the Pipeline, which includes indoctrination (a brutal weeks-long regimen of running, calisthenics, and swimming), dive school, water survival and dunker training (preparing me for emergencies during over-water flights), static-line jump and free-fall courses, and survival and E&E (Escape and Evasion) schools. Additionally, I received over two months of combat medical training (and have since completed basic and intermediate EMT training). All that training is to prepare PJs to make real the search-and-rescue motto: "That Others May Live."

My first rescue operation occurred about six months after completing the Pipeline. Stationed at Nellis Air Force Base in Las Vegas, Nevada, one Saturday afternoon I took a call regarding a possible mission. Rushing to my section, I met with another, more senior, pararescueman, a staff sergeant, and together we reviewed and analyzed the little intelligence we had. What we knew was that a group of civilians in Zion National Park near St. George, Utah, out for a day of climbing and rappelling, had, in setting up their rappelling rig, secured a rope to a small tree above a cliff. One of the climbers, too heavy for the tree, pulled it right out of the ground while rappelling, and he fell about 120 feet to the base of the cliff. Miraculously, the fall did not kill him. Since none of the climbers had radio equipment, several hiked out to a ranger station for help. By the time we finally got the call, several hours had passed.

Quickly getting our gear together, we boarded our HH-60G Pave Hawk helicopter—a combat helicopter often tasked to perform disaster relief, civil search and rescue, and medevac operations—and took off, flying as quickly as possible up to Zion. After a ninety-minute flight, we picked up a park ranger at a ranger station who directed us to the exact site of the accident.

The valley was dangerously narrow, precluding the pilot from hovering close to the ground. The trees growing out of the valley's steeply sloping sides threatened the helicopter's whirling rotors, so we ended up doing about a 140-foot hover above the patient. To make matters worse, the sun had begun to set, so we had to don our night-vision goggles (NVGs)—electro-optical devices affixed to our helmets that amplify existing light in low-light conditions—and fly under "blackout conditions," lights off. Hovering like that over the valley in which the climber had fallen, through the NVG phosphor screen the world seemed a surreal pattern of various shades of green. Climbing out of the hovering aircraft, my partner rode the hoist to the ground in the dark.

Because of the danger the nearby trees posed to the chopper's blades, I remained inside, watching on the left to ensure that our whirling, fifty-three-foot-diameter blades did not hit the jutting trees ten or twelve feet away, while the flight engineer watched on the right. Hovering was pretty damn scary. This was my first "real" rescue mission, and I found myself responsible for making calls to keep the helicopter, moving back and forth in the dark night, and its crew from crashing.

When my partner got to the bottom of the cliff, he found the patient already intubated—a member of the climbing party had crudely, but efficiently, intubated him using the plastic handle of a one-gallon milk container—and properly reintubated him before "packaging" him to be lifted back to the chopper. By now, though, already two and a half hours in flight, we needed to refuel. The clock still ticking, we flew off and quickly refueled. On returning, my partner put the patient on the hoist, and we reeled him in, the motor of the winch just audible in the enveloping din of the chopper's blades. When the hoist reached the cabin door and I'd pulled it in, we climbed away from the hazardous trees and headed for a waiting ambulance while my partner stayed below, both because of the urgency of getting the patient to a hospital and to lead the rest of the climbing party out of the valley.

Because we were still under blackout conditions, I could not appreciate the full extent of the guy's injuries right away. So, once we cleared the trees, I asked the pilot to turn on the interior lights. Removing my NVGs since I could not connect the patient's intubation tube to the oxygen equipment without light, I began blowing through his tube, breathing for him. While I sat leaning over the patient, the lights came on and I jerked backward in shock. The patient's head, because of a basal skull fracture, had blown up like a basketball and blood had run out of his ears and nose. It was much worse than I'd expected.

Putting him on O^2, I checked for a pulse and found none. But, because I was not sure whether this was due to the helicopter's vibrations or because he had no pulse, I erred on the side of caution and began CPR. Because the flight to the ambulance's location was ten, maybe fifteen, minutes, before we arrived, the patient's ribs began to break. Leaning over the patient, arms extended as I performed chest compressions, I felt solid bone sickeningly give way, becoming soft and mushy. Because of the rotors' cacophonous *CHOP-CHOP-CHOP-CHOP,* I could not hear them, but one by one, I felt them crack. The alternative being unacceptable, however, I kept at it until we landed and the ambulance paramedics took over.

After a reflective chopper ride home, I made it my business to find a cold beer and some of my buddies to talk about it. That was one helluva first rescue mission to have done all alone. But, I did it. All those weeks and months of intense training had paid off, and a man who otherwise would have died, lived.

•••

BIOGRAPHY: *Scott Carmack was born in 1967 in Oxnard, California. Carmack enlisted in the Air Force in 1990 after some soul searching and discussions with his father, a retired Navy reservist. Married, he and his wife, Tamara, have three children. Currently assigned to the 38th RQS, 347th Operations Group at Moody AFB in Georgia, Carmack has been a pararescue team member for thirteen years.*

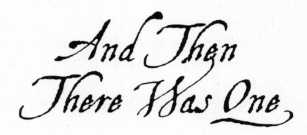

And Then There Was One

By Charles H. Brown

S aipan is about as dissimilar to the arid terrain of Uvalde County, Texas, as a conniving magician could conjure. But the heat found in both places can be stiflingly similar. The humidity for which much of Texas is legendary was something summers in Saipan also offered.

Every able-bodied man I knew in my part of the world had joined the military. So, in December 1942, I enlisted as an apprentice seaman in the U.S. Navy. Trained as a pharmacist's mate, I was going to be a part of the Navy's land forces, which meant that I was attached to the Marine Corps for a while.

August 1945 saw the closing days of World War II, but, of course, at the time, we did not know that. The members of the 2nd Marine Division on Saipan—the "Follow Me" guys—certainly did not. The Japanese were retreating and word came down that we were to canvass Saipan for enemy stragglers, our line corpsmen fanning out to search. My job was to follow them wherever they went. On those nights, my buddies and I followed the line as the island was searched as carefully and uniformly as the terrain and vegetation would allow.

The days were hot, sticky, exhausting, and uncomfortable. The nights were hot, sticky, and even more uncomfortable. Some Pacific island paradise! A beach would have been nice! Our search for Japanese stragglers, unfortunately, occurred across the middle section of the island, where there was no beach. Instead, the terrain was volcanic rock, rugged and rough, in the high ground and dense, tropical vegetation in the valleys of the central part of the island. That made it rough going during the day for sure. The nights were dastardly unpleasant, spent on rocky ground. As the day changed into nighttime colors and the fauna's quartet switched to evening cicada overtures, we tried our best to find a place to make camp that was as smooth as possible. Soft ground was impossible to find. A lot of restless, fitful nights unfolded for most of us. We slept on the ground. We did not sleep in sleeping bags. We did not sleep in tents.

The Division knew there was a high probability for Japanese lying in wait. It was an exercise in high-stakes hide-and-seek. You've played hide-and-seek as kids. You know that your friends are hiding. You just don't know where. As kids you know that the friend hiding is not going to take your life, and still—you hear the squeals of fleeting fright when a hiding friend jumps up and roars at the seeking friend. Your heart races—and this is a game among friends. Imagine that game with enemies and guns. It was a game that went on for days, miles and miles away from family and home. Nerves stood on end unceasingly.

One night, we tried to make our slumber as comfortable as possible. Some of the guys found some high ground that looked to be the best we could do for the night. We clustered in groups. There was a group of six of us and close by another group of six or so. We were all buddies, so there was no special design or order to who slept in which group. As is usual, the duty for watching for the enemy while others slept was determined before we settled into what we derisively called sleep. It is the duty of the first watch to wake the second watch once it is the second watch's turn. The second watch happens at some agreed-upon time around the middle of the night. Irritably, we settled in for what masqueraded as sleep. The first watch completed his stint and moved over to his relief man—our second watchman. As was customary, the first watch shook his relief man to indicate it was his turn.

Who knows what sleep cycle the relief man was in? He bolted upright at being shaken and with his rifle already firing he shrieked, "Nip, Nip, Nip!" I don't know that I ever heard or knew how many shots that fellow fired off that night. Pretty quickly, he was quieted. His frayed nerves and our collective omnipresent fear resulted in a tragic aftermath. The group of six guys that was only a few feet away from the cluster of guys where I slept was left with one. I think it happened quickly. There were six and then there was one, just like that.

It wasn't the enemy. Could any of us have reacted that way that night? In the sweep that we made canvassing for the enemy, I think I saw only two or three. We lost five of our own on that one night in the closing days of the war. We lost five to a nightmare.

How many lives were changed forever that night? The men who died and their families had a quantifiable change to their lives. Equally as vivid and perhaps only a little less measurable, the shooter had his life changed forever. Those of us who were there, just a few feet away and inexplicably spared—we were changed forever. The fellow I wonder about the most, though, was the one who survived from that cluster of six nearby me. Go to sleep with six buddies and wake up the sole survivor. I often wonder about that one.

A lot of lives on both sides were forever changed even in the closing days of World War II. Still, the one I wonder about the most is that one of six who survived. He was just a few feet away from me on that hot, humid, tropical night in August 1945 on that forty-seven-square-mile volcanic island in the Pacific, Saipan.

•••

BIOGRAPHY: *Charles H. Brown was born in Phoenix, Arizona, in 1924. He was raised from his infancy in Uvalde, Texas. Brown entered the U.S. Navy in December 1942 and served as pharmacist's mate, second class. Discharged from the Navy in December 1945, Brown is a retired medical technician who currently resides in Galveston County, Texas.*

Sandstorms and Sweethearts

I first met Specialist (U.S. Army) Don Angle as he walked, holding the hand of one of my dearest friends, Sommer Kader, in our neighborhood; both were still in high school. They'd met while freshmen the second day of school. Sommer noticed a cute guy making his way to campus. Don saw her, his proverbial girl next door. He fell hard and immediately for the brunette with the long curls and exotic eyes. She fell for the sweet-faced blond with the mild disposition. They've been inseparable ever since. I remember how proud Sommer seemed to introduce me to her boyfriend. He firmly shook my hand, never letting his left hand lose grasp with Sommer's.

Today, Don Angle is Sommer's husband. After Donny enlisted in the service in 2000, they decided to marry as soon as they could. So, in August 2001, while on leave for three days, Don said "I do" to Sommer and then promptly returned to duty in Kansas. Shortly thereafter, he left to Kuwait for six months. Sommer stayed in our same neighborhood for much of his tour of duty. Though their contact was limited to occasional cell phone calls and letters, I asked Sommer (okay, badgered Sommer) to ask Donny for a cool story about his experiences in the Middle East for this book. As the deadline approached with my publisher, my hope diminished that I'd get a story from Donny.

Then one Saturday morning, I received the story under unusual circumstances that made me realize the diversity of sacrifice our men and women in uniform make. This particular Saturday, I had slept late, watched cartoons with the kids, sipped my coffee unrushed, and had a big breakfast in the works. I cracked open the eggs and began beating them for imminent scrambling when my cell phone rang. There it was. Sitting on the kitchen counter. Blazing with electronic Mozart. I didn't recognize the number and contemplated not answering it, as I loathed the thought of a disruption on this calm morning of coffee and time with my kids. But at the last moment, I decided to flip the phone on.

"Hello," I said in a perturbed tone. The sound on the other line was grainy—almost like a whooshing in the background of the call. Then I heard the caller.

"Hey, Lynne."

"Who is this?" I demanded, not recognizing the voice on the other end of the receiver.

"It's Don. Don Angle."

I paused in utter disbelief.

Again, I'd been badgering Sommer for weeks to get a story from her husband to tell to me. But I just figured that Sommer could relay something interesting Donny told her in one of their conversations—not actually have him call me!

I knew Donny must have been communicating from overseas, yet I inanely inquired, "Donny? Where are you?"—like he was sitting around the corner in his mother-in-law's kitchen or something.

"Seven miles from the border of Iraq," came his assertive response.

"You're seven miles from the border of Iraq and you're calling me?"

"Yeah. Sommer told me that you needed to talk to me," he politely stated.

We talked and Donny seemed to focus on only one thing: Sommer.

"You know, in our marriage of only a year, Sommer and I have been with each other only two months as husband and wife. I miss her so much. I can stand the 147-degree days here. I can stand the sandstorms and the cots. I just can't stand being away from her for much longer," lamented Donny. "We have wind and sand storms that whip through here every day. I tried to put Sommer's pictures up in the tent. She's beautiful and I just want to be reminded of her, but the sandstorms blow them all down and will destroy them. So I keep a stack of her pictures all together and look at them all the time—whenever I can."

I asked Donny why he serves in the Army when it means being away from Sommer.

He responded authoritatively, "I've always wanted to wear the uniform and serve, and it's really important what I'm doing here. We liberated Kuwait in the Gulf War, and we've had a foothold here for the last ten years. I really believe in keeping Iraq out of this country and letting the Kuwaitis live their lives without fear of invasion and in freedom."

I immediately sensed that Donny also believes in keeping our freedom from terrorism secure, and that the way he accomplishes protecting the United States is by being situated seven miles from the border of Iraq.

When I asked him specifically what's going on, he laconically replied, "I can't tell you anything specific; I won't breach security. I could get court-martialed, and I'm not doing anything to jeopardize returning home to Sommer. But what I can say is that we are well trained. And I know I'll end up back here soon, very soon."

The "very soon" hung in the air; it lingered sickly amidst the satellite connection, and I became aware of the sacrifices that Donny—my dear friend's beloved husband—and his fellow soldiers may need to make if we engage Iraq in war.

Then suddenly, we were out of time, and he "must go back to training." But he asked me to tell Sommer he loves her and relayed that the hardest part of "all this" was on their anniversary. "I couldn't call her at all on August 19; I couldn't even call to say 'Happy Anniversary' on the day we wed."

Recently, Sommer and Donny's families gathered at Sommer's childhood home, where her mother held a going-away party for her—she was leaving for Fort Riley, Kansas, to set up their base home and await Donny's return from the Gulf. After ten months' separation out of twelve months of marriage, they would soon find themselves together. I brought a little something for Sommer from a popular lingerie store. The box contained items delicate and romantic. I just figured that Donny—who called me from Kuwait at the behest of his wife, endured 147-degree heat for months, lived in a tent during miserable and frequent sandstorms, suffered the separation from his new bride, and even potentially risked his life so that my children and I may sleep a little more soundly and feel a little safer in this war on terrorism—well, Donny deserved to finally celebrate his anniversary a few months late, looking upon his wife wearing something NOT in desert camouflage.

To all those "Don Angles" out there who leave their own families to protect ours, thank you.

...

BIOGRAPHY: *Don Angle was born in 1977 in Sacramento, California, and lived most of his life in neighboring areas. He enlisted in the Army in January 2000 and iscurrently a Specialist (E-4) in the infantry. Angle plans to attend Ranger school and hopes to build a career in the service by completing his degree and serving as an officer in the future. In the summer of 2001, Angle married his high school sweetheart, Sommer Kader. The couple makes their home at Fort Riley, Kansas. Angle's story, incidentally, came by cell phone as he sat only seven miles from the border of Iraq protecting Kuwait and fought the war on terrorism.*

We Were Tired!

By Robert Clark
as told to Shauna Seymour

My combat experience was in the Philippines fighting the Japanese, in World War II. I was a lieutenant in the Army in charge of a platoon of about forty men when I started out on this particular campaign. By the time this particular campaign was over, half of my men had been either killed or badly wounded.

Rather than dwell on some of the more unpleasant happenings of World War II, and there were plenty of them, I will tell you about an experience that was rather funny.

My platoon and I were gathered in a small circle in an open space about two hundred yards behind the enemy lines. As we were to move up on the enemy the next day, I was giving instructions as to what they were to do. Suddenly, we heard the roar of an airplane approaching at a very low altitude. We looked up to see that it was one of our own bombers, a B-25, hit by antiaircraft fire and in flames and crashing. Then, to our horror, we saw a bomb break loose from the plane's undercarriage and come plummeting straight down at us.

Now, nobody likes to be blown up by a bomb, and it is especially embarrassing when that bomb is coming from one of your own planes. I will tell you now that my men were very brave, but there is a saying that "Discretion is the better part of valor," and my men and I took that advice to heart.

We ran and scattered like scared jackrabbits. The "bomb" landed right where, a few seconds before, we had been standing. Only it wasn't a bomb. It was a tire that had burned away from the plane and fell. The tire hit the earth, bounced high in the air, and continued to bounce and careen down the hill, sending my fellow soldiers scattering pell-mell for safety.

Normally, after such a scary experience you would expect everyone to be busy thanking their lucky stars that it had been only a tire and not a bomb. But there was a continuing drama going on. We all looked up to watch the plane as it continued toward the hills behind us, heading for a flaming crash and certain death for the crew of the craft.

But then we witnessed a near miracle. As we watched, one by one, the white puffs of parachutes opened below the plane. We counted as five chutes opened and five crewmen floated down to land safely on the ground. Only the pilot was still with the plane. It continued on, lower and lower, flames still spurting from its engines, and then suddenly it was gone, out of our sight.

It was very quiet for several minutes, and then we heard a loud explosion and saw flames and smoke rise up where the plane had gone down. We watched with mixed feelings. We were glad that we had not been "bombed." We were happy for the five men who parachuted safely from that plane, but we all also felt saddened for that brave pilot who had gone down with his craft. The fact that he had stayed at the controls made it possible for his crew to save themselves. Is this a sad ending?

It should have been, but we learned the next day that that pilot was not only brave, but he was also skillful. He had landed his huge, burning plane, without wheels, on the ridge of a hill, and after landing it, he had calmly climbed out and walked away, completely unscathed. I never learned what happened to the pilot, but I hope he received a well-deserved medal. I do know he left behind five very appreciative airmen and a bunch of paratroopers who were very grateful that he had dropped a tire on them instead of a bomb.

•••

BIOGRAPHY: *Robert Clark was born in Kokomo, Indiana, in 1921. Clark decided to join the Army soon after the Japanese attack on Pearl Harbor. After the war, he went to college on the GI Bill and taught music in high school and computer science at junior college. He has two sons, Brice and Scott Clark, and four stepdaughters, Linda, Susan, Colleen, and Janelle. He is married to Janet Clark. Now retired, the octogenarian writes and directs plays.*

My Little Black Book

By Mark Finlayson

I f you've ever been in the military, you probably remember the scene vividly—walking through the doors of MEPS (the Military Entrance Processing Station), realizing your life is about to change forever. Mine certainly did, in two very profound ways; one expected and one totally unexpected but far more important.

My passage through MEPS occurred on April 14, 1987, as a very young eighteen-year-old, totally focused on becoming a United States Marine. I always knew I would go to college and pursue a different career, but first I had to fulfill a compelling personal desire to be part of an elite team. I wanted to be the best of the best, to challenge myself, to create a permanent change in who I was. Yet, at the same time, I didn't really know who I wanted to be or what I was looking for or what needed changing; I just knew I wanted to be a part of something perfect, pure, and I thought I'd attain that in the Marines.

That spring day, my recruiter escorting me to the seventh floor of the MEPS building at Broad and Cherry Streets in Philadelphia, I was surprised to find someone from The Gideons International standing outside the building entrance. The well-dressed man was distributing black, soft-cover, pocket-edition New Testaments—for whatever reason they did not have the green-covered Bibles normally given to military personnel—to each of us passing through those doors on a one-way trip to a new life. At that time, I was not very "religious." However, having been raised to respect Godly things, I politely thanked the man and, while others quickly discarded their Bibles in the first accessible garbage can, stowed mine in my gear. Giving it no further thought (being focused on the next thirteen weeks of recruit training at Parris Island), I crossed the building's threshold, taking the first step from being a civilian individual to becoming a member of a military team.

The first Sunday in my new home, located in the middle of the Broad River in South Carolina, the drill instructors (DIs) explained that we were allowed to go to church for two hours if we so chose. Quite honestly, I really wasn't interested in church, and a two-hour service sounded painful, but when I heard the chapel was air-conditioned and DI-free, I decided definitively to attend. Meanwhile, according to our DIs, my platoon had a record number of "untrainables." The DIs' definition of an "untrainable" was a recruit from Philadelphia (my home), New Jersey, or the New York area. Our untrainable count was twenty-one out of a total platoon population of seventy-seven. At this point of boot camp, I was the platoon guide, though I didn't feel much like the leader of seventy-seven recruits. Young and impressionable, I found myself often looking up to the older and more hardened recruits from the inner-city communities of the Bronx, Brooklyn, Queens, Staten Island, and Jersey City. These guys were my best friends in the platoon, and I viewed them as older brothers.

In church, though, it was many of these same untrainables that so struck me as I watched them crooning like canaries Gospel songs I had never heard before. That was the first time I realized you could both love God and be "cool." These guys were tough, not to be messed with; yet they were singing out to a Lord I did not know. The scene stuck with me and made me think. And even though I still didn't crack open that little Bible, I began to keep it in my left breast pocket, the pocket that also included the USMC insignia.

Boot camp came and went, as did advanced training and fleet duty, first in South Carolina, then Oklahoma, Philadelphia, and, finally, San Diego. Each was home for a time, then little more than a memory. Wherever I went, though, that little black Book always seemed to get packed up, brought along, and placed back in my left breast pocket. As you might have guessed, there came a day when I actually opened it, a day when life just seemed overwhelming and too difficult to handle. So, turning to page one, I began to read. For the first time, I read words that were so important that a man—whom I neither knew nor would ever see again—took time to see that every wide-eyed kid walking through the doors of my MEPS station received a copy.

It was years later, though, that I came to understand the meaning of those words, why they were so important, and even how they were actually working in my life just by their presence in my gear and breast pocket. I have since read many different translations of the entire Bible, front to back, over and again. However, that first pocket-sized Bible with the black cover still accompanies me everywhere in the glove compartment of my car. The pages are a bit tattered and the cover is worn, but the words of that book are forever etched within the heart and mind of this Marine.

Recently, pondering the influence of that gift from the Gideons so long ago, I realized something special about the workings of God in my life. In my parents' house hang four pictures—one each of me, my mother, my father, and my sister. Under each is a gold plaque inscribed with each person's name, the name's meaning, and a scripture verse. Mine reads: "Mark, 'Mighty Warrior,' I Timothy 6–12, the Lord's call to fight the good fight of faith." I came suddenly to appreciate the significance of my name, the verse, the Marines, and that little Bible, all working together. I had joined the Corps believing in my destiny to serve my country as a warrior, fighting for freedom. That Bible, given to me at the beginning of my military life, its message the birth of my spiritual life, was a quiet prophesy that I would become a Christian warrior, too. While I had chosen the Marines to be changed forever, God had chosen me to be changed for good. Ooh Rah!

•••

BIOGRAPHY: *Mark Finlayson was born in 1968 in Philadelphia, Pennsylvania. He spent six years enlisted in the Marines and Marine Corp Reserves, attaining the rank of sergeant (E-5) in less than three years. A graduate of Temple University, Finlayson is an educator and a technology consultant living in the suburbs of Philadelphia. The father of one daughter, Finlayson is the author of the children's book* Front Frog Fred and Back Frog Jack.

The Cane Map

By Jill Labbe

No one can say for sure how my father, Boyd Lee Grubaugh, got the nickname "Dan." My mother thinks it was a shortened version of "Dirty-Neck Dan," a handle tagged on him by crew members commenting on how grungy his flight suit got after hours of training exercises. He made his debut, at a robust twelve pounds, on March 14, 1918. As described by his mother, he was round faced with a long upper lip; his eyes had a sporty look and his shoulders were very broad. His dark brown hair swirled in a double crown, which he kept under control by cutting one close. My grandmother once wrote that Southerners say a double crown is a sign that you'll eat your bread in two kingdoms. Daddy Dan ate in many after he volunteered for the Army Air Corps. He had enrolled at State University in Bowling Green, Ohio, with an inclination toward pre-med courses. With so many friends volunteering for war service as pilots, however, Daddy Dan felt pangs to join them. He did not re-enter college for the spring term in 1941 and was sworn into service.

Prior to being one of the pioneer pilots of the B-29 Superfortress in the China-Burma-India theater, Daddy Dan was an instructor at Ellington Field in Texas. He returned to the states after the mission detailed below to become chief test pilot at Edwards Air Force Base in California. Lt. Col. Boyd Lee Grubaugh would die there during a test flight in 1958. As my grandmother wrote in a memoir to his children, "We understand it was quick and merciful, and in all honor. He was a Praying Pilot." He is buried in Arlington National Cemetery.

I never heard stories about the B-29 Superfortress from my father, even though he was among the first pilots to fly Boeing's revolutionary aircraft into combat. He died in a crash at Edwards Air Force Base when my twin brother and I were only two. Research—that indispensable tool of a journalist—turned up information that the B-29 was considered an ideal weapon to fulfill the War Department's mission for the Twentieth Air Force: the application of a new refinement of global warfare. The Super Fort's remarkable range was particularly suited for the long over-water flight required to attack the Japanese homeland from bases in China.

Before my birth, my father, Capt. Boyd Lee Grubaugh, spent ten months in the China-Burma-India theater after having arrived in India in March of 1944. By piecing together information from letters he wrote home to my aunts and uncles, along with official Army Air Corps/Air Force documents, I learned that he was part of the Twentieth Bomber Command whose mission it was to pound the Japanese city of Yawata, announcing to the world that a new era in American air superiority had dawned.

But twenty-six-year-old Daddy Dan's participation in those June 1944 strikes against Japanese industrial targets was cut short by flak and a thunderstorm.

"As we were coming off the target at Yawata, Japan, flak knocked out our No. 1 engine and put both our rear gun turrets out of operation," my father told a reporter for the Santa Ana Army Air Base newspaper in March of 1945. "A Japanese fighter then attacked from below and raked the ship from stem to stern, seriously wounding the top-turret gunner and ruining the flight instruments." Within the hour, the gunner was dead. There was little time then to mourn. Job 1 was repairing the instruments so that the rest of the crew could be saved.

"We really ran into trouble when we hit very rough weather," Daddy Dan continued in the report. "The big ship was thrown violently about by the storm; we hit one terrific updraft that tossed the B-29 over on its back. I got the plane back on an even keel by flipping it into a dive at 450 miles per hour. "When we pulled out at 7,000 feet, I discovered that I had no control over the plane. The violent maneuver and dive had either sprung the wings or ripped fabric off the elevators, making control impossible. There was nothing to do but to order the crew to bail out." According to Air Force reports, my father was the last man to leave the plane when he jumped at 7,000 feet. He watched as the Super Fort crashed into the side of a mountain. The plane wasn't the only thing to hit mountain; the pilot smacked into one on his landing, fracturing a knee. He hid out until daylight and, after making a crutch from a small tree, started out to seek help.

That crutch would become a legend in the family and a lifesaver for future Hump pilots. Throughout his thirty-day journey around China, aided by various farmers, Daddy Dan would have the friendlies carve the symbols for their villages into the cane. It would become a roadmap for future pilots seeking safety and help.

One farmer constructed a litter and had my father transported by two coolies. In one village, he and two crew members who found the same community were feted to a banquet fit for royality—or liberating American pilots.

"The Chinese gave us a 24-course dinner, including such delicacies as 100-year-old eggs," Daddy told the Crossroads reporter. "It was a five-hour meal and every man of importance in the village made a toast to us. We were the first American flyers they had ever seen.

"The following day, the local mandarin provided us with coolie bearers to continue the journey. These bearers carried us 40 miles in 10 hours over rugged mountain trails and we finally reached an advanced 14th Air Force base."

Two more of the B-29's crew members were at this base, which was within five minutes' flying time of a Japanese airdrome. The survivors stayed at the airfield for three weeks before a C-47 could slip in to return them to their home base.

My dad's leg suffered from the lack of medical attention, and he was returned to the States for further treatment. In later years, people said that when he was tired, his lameness became more noticeable.

But more than his leg suffered from the experience. In his role as the ship's captain, he took the responsibility for his crew to heart. Years later, he still mourned the loss of that unnamed gunner. In her memoir to her grandchildren, Ada Grubaugh wrote that Boyd "could not forget nor discuss it. Just said, 'I can't stand civilians; one question and my grief lies out on the table. So I'll never leave the Air Corps.'"

•••

BIOGRAPHY: *Boyd Lee "Dan" Grubaugh was born on March 14, 1918, the third of six children born to William and Ada Grubaugh of Ohio. He volunteered for Army Air Corps' cadet training program and was sworn into service on his twenty-third birthday. After the war, he returned to the States and ultimately became chief test pilot at Edwards Air Force Base in California. It was there that Lt. Col. Boyd Lee Grubaugh, USAF, would die on June 16, 1958, during a test flight in the arid skies above the Mojave Desert, leaving behind a wife and three children.*

Almost Dead Again

By Paul Eugene Rominger

as told to Lynne Rominger

The day I was shot down and then ultimately captured and detained in a concentration camp as a POW, my crew and I were assigned an F model B-17, though we initially were dubbed supernumerary for the mission. *Supernumerary* meant that we would go on the mission only if another plane proved inoperable at takeoff. As the neophyte flyers just in to Foggia, Italy, by way of Greenland, the plan seemed reasonable enough. Send the experienced pilots in first—and the "green" guys only if really needed, right?

Ominously, earlier in the day, a friend of mine actually said, "Paul, I hope all the other planes take off okay, because that plane they've assigned to you is the old, beat-up F model, and it won't make it back." My buddy's words echoed in the back of my mind and an uneasiness descended on me when I learned my crew was taking the place of another plane that had to abort the mission. Indeed, later that day— the day of my first combat mission out of flight school—my friend's unfortunate prophecy came true. But, although the bomber may not have made it back over the Alps and home to Italy, by the end of my inaugural flight over foreign soil, I would have escaped death three times.

The mission started and virtually finished without incident; we had bombed the Skoda Works at Pilsen, Czechoslovakia, and were on our way back to Italy flying at thirty-two thousand feet when suddenly my group of planes—and my plane in particular—began taking flak (antiaircraft fire). I heard a *WHUMP* and then a loud crack as the air-bursting artillery shells hit and knew our troubles were just beginning. Suddenly a tremendous roar of cold wind engulfed the cabin. A piece of shrapnel literally blew a large hole in the floor of the plane between my legs and another hole in the area just above my head. I curbed my panic while, at the same time, feeling relief that I hadn't had my legs crossed during the first assault, when another hole appeared—this one in the number-three engine.

Oil began pouring out. No oil, no running engine. My crew and I were clearly in desperate circumstances at this point, when I tried to feather the prop. But the beat-up F model that my buddy had warned me about had a different prop/hydraulic system than the new G models that I'd learned to fly in. The oil pressure for feathering is the same as the engine hydraulic pressure on the F model (unlike on the newer G models, which had a separate system for feathering) and engine pressure dropped so suddenly that the prop would not feather. Meanwhile, the number-two engine was on fire, and the number-one engine had also stopped. We lost speed and altitude fast.

Amidst the silent Hail Marys and Lord's prayers, I told the crew to bail out. One of them, probably shocked about the quick change in our previously placid flight, questioned me, saying, "Bail out, sir!?" I reaffirmed that it was a good idea. After the entire crew had parachuted from the descending plane, I finally made my way to the bomb bay and dropped through, looking forward to a silky parachute ride to solid ground. But, my problems were just beginning.

At least with the antiflak coming in the cockpit, I hadn't anticipated or had time to think about impending death—but on the other occasions, the fear of my precarious mortality loomed closely. On both of the other occasions I thought or knew I was going to be killed within a few seconds.

Remember when I dropped through the bomb bay, looking forward to the silky parachute flight to solid ground? Well, when I bailed out, my backpack parachute didn't open when I pulled the ripcord. I was plunging to the ground without protection at a rate of over 160 feet per second. Desperately, I tried to reach the chute cover on my back, but the heavy winter flying suit made it impossible. As crazy as it may sound, in momentary resignation to my fate, I spread my arms and legs to cushion the shock of hitting the ground. By that time, I had probably fallen to about ten thousand feet from a bail-out altitude of twenty-three thousand feet. Perhaps the extra oxygen at my new altitude stimulated my next thought, but more likely a miracle was afoot and God was giving me another chance and planting ingenuity in a sort of MacGyver way. At any rate, I figured that if I tucked myself tightly together in a fetal position and tumbled in the air, the wind might catch the chute flaps from a different angle and blow them open. It worked! As I tumbled in a dizzying circle, I saw a white flash of chute, which jerked me into an upright position with such violence that I thought I'd broken my neck, and suffered weeks after with pain. But I was still alive! I looked up at the canopy with gratitude for a moment and then beyond the canopy I noticed several small white dots—my crew members whose chutes had opened without incident or delay.

But my peace at the parachute opening soon disintegrated with a distant roar getting louder. Here is where my third brush with death began. I looked up beyond the canopy and soon saw our plummeting plane in a tight spiral, its number-four engine getting louder and more deafening as it headed right toward me! I was certain that the plane's path and mine would cross in about five seconds and once again felt the clock ticking in a race for life. I pulled almost hysterically at the shroud lines to steer out of the descending bomber's path, but to no avail; thousands of pounds of metal continued to plummet directly toward me. I felt like a bug about to splat into an oncoming windshield. The plane was in a vertical bank just opposite me as I looked at it head-on and saw clearly into the front window where I had been sitting just a few minutes before. But instead of hitting me, miraculously the huge B-17 passed less than a few feet under me.

Fog serenely hugged the wooded area in which I safely landed. The chute even draped over a small tree, which allowed me to touch the ground very gently. After burying the chute, I left the area in case someone had seen my descent. As I ran through the woods en route to Switzerland and safety, I heard what I thought was an unusual-sounding engine. I stopped to try to determine from where the noise was coming and evaluate my security; I discovered that the sound was not an engine but instead the pounding of my own heart! As I continued my walk in the direction of Switzerland, I came to the edge of the woods and looked across an open field to a peaceful farm scene. I stepped out into the open field and there, only fifteen feet to my right, was a German soldier with his back to me and a rifle on his shoulder. Needless to say, I quietly turned around and left the field. Only after the sun went down and darkness descended did I attempt my flight by foot to the Alps and back to Italy. Later that night, I pulled pine boughs from a tree and put them on the ground for a makeshift pallet and slept, thankful that I had lived. My journey home, unfortunately, was to be delayed even longer than I anticipated.

As the sun rose the next morning, farmers saw me before I awakened. Soon, a mob converged upon me from all directions. They held shovels, rakes, hoes, and other tools as they rushed toward me. Interestingly, I remember thinking how much these Germans looked like the neighbor farmers and friends I had known in Ohio growing up. I was, quite frankly, amazed at the similarity between the enemy and myself. I didn't know it at the time, but the part of Germany where I was captured was near the area from which my ancestors had migrated to the United States in 1742. Though the local sheriff took me to jail, the next day I was escorted toward the German interrogation center at Rhein-Main. Traveling on foot, by car, and by train, the trip took days.

I was one of about thirty POWs. When we finally exited the train at our last destination, as we marched through the streets to the interrogation center, the civilians spit at us and one called out "Neger und Juden!" (Interestingly, only two years later, I would be back in Germany on the same street and the civilians stepped off the sidewalks to let me pass.)

Before we were segregated at the interrogation center, the POWs had a brief moment to actually speak to one another. I immediately sought out one of my crew who ironically asked if "I'd known who it was that almost got hit by our plane." Needless to say, I was able to give him a firsthand account of the near hit.

After the interrogation, we ended up in a POW camp—very much unlike the comfortable accommodations of Stalag 13 of *Hogan's Heroes*. My ordeal lasted six months and included many more harrowing situations, including starvation and hiking miles during sieges in blizzard conditions, before we were liberated. Through it all, I never gave up hope. I just figured that God had given me the wits and perseverance to defy death three times in one day, and I never lost faith in our troops and their eventual success. Later in my detainment, an Army major was captured and brought to the camp. He confirmed that the Allies were close. We all knew then that "our flag was still there" and would arrive flying high proclaiming liberty.

I don't think there was a dry eye in the camp when, within days, we did see the American flag raised over Mooseburg. I will never forget the emotion and love of country we all felt at that moment. Soon General Patton, pearl-handled revolvers and all, rode through the main gate of our camp on a tank! He was appalled by our living conditions but said clearly that "the Germans are paying for it!" Ten days later, my own brother, Don, a chief mate in the Merchant Marines, transported me home to the United States from France on his ship. I was finally home sweet home.

●●●

BIOGRAPHY: *Paul Rominger was born in Youngstown, Ohio, on January 16, 1922. Rominger graduated from Chaney High School in 1940, and then* moved to San Diego, California, where he worked as a sheet metal assembler in an aircraft company before joining the U.S. Army Air Corps in 1943. He retired at the rank of major from the U.S. Air Force on December 31, 1962, with twenty-two and a half years of service. He then worked for eleven years with the Planning Department of the City of San Jose, California. He now lives in Mobile, Alabama, finally in full retirement, except for occasional work at the tourist attraction known as Bellingrath Gardens.

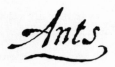

Ants

By Thomas Hartman

I'd been in Panama less than three weeks, and with my unit only two weeks, when I found myself rucking-up for a major field exercise. The old-timers in Charlie Company, 2nd Battalion, 187th Light Airborne Infantry Regiment, told me every horror story imaginable about jungle operations: scorpions in your boots, howler monkeys screaming like the damned, killer bees, tarantulas crawling over you, poison tree frogs that kill on touch, poison snakes that hunt you, poison snakes that hang from trees and strike you, nonpoisonous snakes that crush you, vampire bats, spiders that lay eggs in your skin, walking off cliffs at night, impalement upon black palm, wait-a-minute vines, jungle rot, brain fever, and leprosy. I thought I knew them all.

Eight days into the field exercise, we were scheduled for one last daytime assault on a fixed position, followed by a hot meal and truck ride back to the barracks. During the previous eight days, I'd already experienced maneuvering in ten-foot-high grass, neck-deep swamp, and triple-canopy jungle. I'd seen scorpions, tarantulas, killer bees, and even a small boa constrictor. By the third night, I managed to put my fears to rest and fall asleep seconds after my watch ended. This final assault would involve firing off a lot of ammo and use certain specialty weapons, including the 90mm recoilless rifle (think World War II bazooka) and the M203 grenade launcher.

The assault went well. I could taste the promised hot meal and feel the cool breeze from the truck ride. I could also taste the first of many cold beers I'd planned to consume at the NCO Club that night. I soon found out, though, that "the trucks are on the way" and "a hot meal is in the works" are the infantry equivalent to "the check is in the mail." Orders came down that we were to ruck-up and E&E (escape and evade) to a rendezvous point five klicks (kilometers) back. The punishment for being captured would be the loss of weekend privileges.

I'd already quickly learned that five klicks in the jungle is a lot farther than a five-klick hump along a surface road. Terrain, weather, and daylight affect pace and distance. This was very hilly, triple-canopy jungle; it had just rained; and daylight was beginning to fade. Movement at night in the jungle is not just difficult, it is brutal. Under triple-canopy jungle at night, there is no light. You can literally wave your hand in front of your face and not see it. Even night-vision devices do not work, and you cannot use a flashlight, of course, because it would give away your position. To stay in contact with your unit, you have to keep your hand on the rucksack of the person ahead of you, while the point man uses a self-illuminating compass to follow an azimuth. If he runs into a tree, he steps around it and continues. (There are a lot of problems with this method. On a subsequent mission, I saw [heard, actually] a guy on point and the guy behind him walk over a small cliff. Another time, two platoons were completely separated because a man had grabbed a branch instead of the man's rucksack in front of him and fallen asleep standing up.) Anyway, under such conditions, our five-klick E&E evolved into fourteen hours of misery. For a squad mate and me, the misery began in earnest around 0200 hours.

We'd been moving slowly and unsteadily about eight hours. Between humping a sixty-five-pound rucksack, slipping repeatedly in the mud, getting caught on wait-a-minute vines, and being eaten alive by mosquitoes, everyone had a major "case of the ass" (bad attitude). We'd just stopped (for the hundredth time) on the side of a hill, when

I heard a strange sound, like water running out of a faucet. I whispered to my squad mate in front of me, "What the f—— is that? There wasn't anything there a minute ago."

He responded in kind: "I don't f——ing know!"

Then, I noticed a strange smell—very acrid, unlike anything I'd smelled before—and began to feel sweat running up (yes, up) my legs. At that point, I'd had enough. I pulled out my flashlight and turned it on, a major military no-no. Pointing the beam down, I saw my pants moving, though my legs were not. Standing in the middle of a very large ant hive, we'd interrupted their slumber. In front of me, my buddy, yelling "Ants!" ran straight into a tree. The next moment, it seemed like my ankles, legs, and buttocks were dipped in fire; all the ants had both bitten and stung simultaneously. Screaming in a very unmanly fashion, I ran, then felt someone grab me and throw me to the ground. I started rolling and smacking my legs frantically, while another guy helped the first one pin me down and a third quickly undid my fatigues, and they proceeded to pick the ants off, one by one.

These were not ordinary ants; they were cutter ants—the kind featured on nature specials, usually shown carrying leaves through the jungle. Larger than carpenter ants, about one-half-inch long, they cannot merely be slapped off. Each must be pulled off because they grab skin with their pincers, then sting with a poisoned barb.

After they picked all of the ants off of us, the medic gave me and my buddy Benedryl and the whole platoon took a short rest before rucking-up again and marching for another eight hours. The pain was phenomenal. My head was ringing, my skin on fire, my muscles on the brink of cramping, and I was very woozy. I later learned we had over one hundred bites, mine all over my ankles, legs, buttocks, and genitals.

We made it to the rendezvous point around 0800 hours, the trucks sitting in the clearing, first and second platoons eating a hot breakfast. They'd waited all night for us, having marched out to the rendezvous point in about four hours without incident.

As I was sitting down for chow, my platoon sergeant approached me. I had a great deal of respect for this man; he'd seen combat and had been a very patient teacher. "Hartman," he said. "I understand you are new to the Army, new to the Airborne, and new to the bush. However, you need to think on a couple of things. First, all our training is in preparation for the real deal, combat. Second, the habits you acquire in training you will carry with you into combat. This morning, you jeopardized the entire platoon. Do you know how?"

"Yes, Sergeant," I said. "I turned on my flashlight and could have exposed our position to the enemy."

"That's partially correct," he replied. "It was your first mistake. Your second was screaming and yelling."

Incredulous, I thought, "How was I supposed to not yell?"

He saw it in my face. "You are a paratrooper in the United States Army. You are one of the elite, and the Army and I expect you to behave that way. I don't know about you, but I'd be embarrassed if I acted like that. In addition, the pain of those stings would've been nothing to the pain you'd have felt if a single platoon member was wounded or killed by your actions. I am speaking from personal experience."

I looked him in the eye and said, "It will not happen again."

"Good enough." Before walking away, he added, "You should be very proud of the way you handled yourself for the rest of the march; you did not complain and you did not quit."

That conversation was a turning point for me. I realized I had to be a soldier. Throughout basic training, advanced infantry training, and airborne school, I'd been playing soldier. During the rest of my tour in Panama, I had encounters with killer bees, vampire bats, fire ants, and heat stroke, but I never made those mistakes again.

•••

BIOGRAPHY: *Thomas Hartman was born in 1965 in Philadelphia, Pennsylvania, and grew up there. Tom entered the U.S. Army after high school and served his country for three years. After being honorably discharged in 1986, Tom graduated from Temple University and is now co-owner of a home-restoration business. He and wife, Patty, are the proud parents of two.*

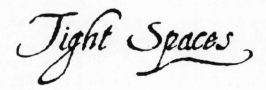

Tight Spaces

By Edward William Hippo
as told by Melissa Hippo

December, in the south of France. The weather was cold, but not as bad as back home in Pennsylvania. I was a sergeant in an infantry unit, with only three men still with me from the day I first landed. The rest were replacements who seemed nice enough, but with the war nearly over, I finally had to worry about myself and getting home. Sometimes I tired of nursemaiding kids who should have been running up and down the football fields of Some State U instead of trying to keep from being killed or wounded on a battlefield thousands of miles from home. Occasionally, we would see an officer, but often we didn't see any brass for days at a time. On this day, however, our lieutenant happened to be with us. He was all right, but an officer is an officer, and we were not too terribly fond of most of them. Low on food and everything else a soldier needed, we were waiting at a cross-roads for gasoline, rations, and ammunition, everyone talking about the French women who, had they smelled me then, would certainly have been as fond of me as I was of officers. I'd have given a month's pay for some booze to drink at that moment.

When it was finally time to move, I had a feeling that things were going to get much worse. Like the rest of the men, I wished I had a house to sleep in that night. Moving over several hills, we fortuitously came to what was left of a farmhouse and barn. Though the Germans burned or destroyed buildings so we could not use them for cover, this one happened to be in decent shape. I told my men to keep their eyes open moving in, and to be careful not to shoot me (the new guys—always "trying" to see more action—would pretty much shoot at anything). The farmhouse sat some fifty yards away, and the sun was beginning to set. The house was typical of those dotting that war-ravaged region. Built of stone, a few shreds of curtains waved from some of the windows. We could've used a bed and some clean sheets, of course, but I may as well have wished for a steak dinner and some cold beer. We had to settle for a roof over our heads. Moving toward the farmhouse, I suddenly—I don't know why—was struck by the random thought that Germans didn't want to die any more than I did.

Once inside, we settled down and pooled together our K rations to see whether we had enough food for all of us. The new guys, still hasty, as always ate too fast. Soon after eating, we were off to sleep—war had taught me to sleep at a moment's notice and in increments. A couple of guards out front kept watch, the new recruits alternating two hours on and two hours off.

From the welcome refuge of sleep, Smitty (damn it!) woke me and ruined my dream—I had been in a house with a beautiful woman and plenty of food and wine. He told me that he'd found a cache of wine in the root cellar under the house. To my dismay, though, there was also a young civilian woman hiding there; it was less agreeable in real life than it had been in my dream. The Germans who'd recently quickly pulled out had left her behind. She was very happy to see me. Right after I'd taken personal responsibility for the cache of food and wine, I learned why the Germans had left so fast. An artillery barrage suddenly rained down all around us. When the shells came in, we did the only thing we could—we got horizontal right quick and prayed.

Beams crashed down on the floor upstairs. It was confusing, but I knew we were trapped and the Germans were pulling the noose tight. The next shell landed very close; my world became cloudy and dark, and I could no longer move my legs. The French girl stopped moving at all. I yelled and yelled, but no one answered. Then, the next voices I heard were speaking German! I knew I was in deep trouble. In my pitch-black, closed-in world, I'd lost all sense of time. My back—and every other part of me for that matter—ached. I wanted to cry out, to get out of there. "Some coal miner's son I am," I thought. "Where is my strength?" I wondered, until, finding that if I thought of home or my girl I didn't want to scream, I located its source.

Some time later—I couldn't tell how much time had passed—I heard voices yelling again. This time, though, one of them had a New York accent. I later learned the full story. My men had regrouped at the barn, deciding, I guess, that they missed their old sarge after all. The German troops I had heard talking apparently had tired of their own artillery shooting at them, and when they left, my boys came back and dug me out from under the timbers that had me pinned down, though, thankfully, with little injury.

Ever since that incident, I have hated tight spaces, though my love for wine has never faded.

•••

BIOGRAPHY: *Edward William Hippo was the fifth son of Pennsylvania coal miners. He was the only child in the family to actually finish high school. After graduation at the beginning of World War II, he enlisted in the Army. A rifle-man in the European theater, Hippo also drove one of Patton's personal jeeps. Fond of his Lucky Strikes, Edward William Hippo died of lung cancer when only fifty-three years old.*

Three Brothers and a War

By Eldon Johnson

as told to his grandson, Nicholas Depner

The 1944 reunion of the three Johnson brothers from Kansas City during World War II should, by all odds, have never taken place. Two brothers served in the Army two hundred miles apart, one in India, the other in Burma, and the third served aboard ship in the Navy. But sometimes miracles (and a little ingenuity) can make all the difference.

When his ship received orders over the radio early in the morning on a beautiful subtropical day, Navy Lieutenant (Senior Grade) Lamont R. Johnson stood in disbelief on the bridge of his liberty ship. Could they have really been ordered into the nearest Indian port? He immediately saw in this his golden opportunity to reconnect with at least one, if not both, of his brothers fighting in India and Burma.

After his ship docked in the then-Indian port of Karachi, however, the mistake had been realized; these orders were intended not for Lamont's ship, but rather a different ship also steaming in the waters of the Indian Ocean. Since it would take at least three days to provision the ship for its return to duty, Lamont took it upon himself to set out for the local Air Transport Command office, where he explained his situation and gave the last known location of his brothers. All he needed now was permission from the Navy commandant in Karachi, which, unfortunately, was flatly and unceremoniously denied.

Returning to the ship disheartened, Lamont thought to himself, "What the hell? I have just as much rank as he does!" With that in mind, he returned to the Air Transport Command office where a high-priority "mail courier" pass was written for him. Mail courier pass in hand, Lamont boarded a C-47 cargo transport aircraft, which putted along at a frustratingly slow 120 mph, pogo-sticking its way across the Indian subcontinent.

Lamont's last cross-country junket stop was Assam, India, where his youngest brother, First Lieutenant fighter pilot Eldon Johnson, was visiting a friend in the local military hospital. A khaki uniform—clad Army nurse came rushing into the hospital room excitedly addressing Eldon: "Johnny! Johnny! Your brother is here!"

Since Eldon's middle brother, Linden, frequently made visits, the pilot dismissed the nurse's shouts, assuming Linden, passing through, was making a typical stopover. "No, no," the nurse continued loudly, "not Linden! It's your brother from the NAVY!" Ten minutes later, Lamont stepped into the room in his dress whites, an impressive, if ill-conceived, gesture in the mucky, humid Indian jungle.

Eldon was overjoyed to see his sibling. But there wasn't time to hang out; they wanted to get to Linden. The two brothers piled into a jeep for the rough and bumpy forty-mile drive back to Eldon's base. While there, they wasted no time in contacting Eldon's commanding officer. Sympathetic to the brothers' request, he approved their request to board yet another flight, this time to the city of Myitkyina, Burma, two hundred miles to the south over steep, rugged mountain ranges.

The following morning, travel passes in hand, Lamont and Eldon climbed into the C-47 transport—loaded expressively with empty coffins on their final journey before "seeing action" in the war. Upon arrival at seven o'clock the next morning on the allied landing strip in Myitkyina, the two brothers were more than happy to remove themselves from the gruesome transport.

Not until they stepped foot off the C-47 did they realize that these wooden boxes were, in fact, destined for Myitkyina, too; the city had been under siege for no less than eighty-four days. The brothers surveyed the air base, a quagmire of mud from the heavy monsoon rains and the high traffic on the roads. Dotting the area, temporary shelters—tents over waterlogged foxholes—bespoke the intense fighting and nighttime Japanese artillery barrages on the air base.

Weaving among parked P-40 Flying Tiger fighters, C-47 "Gooney Bird" transports, and jeeps, Lamont and Eldon made their way from the parking stand of the cargo transport. Intelligence officer for the 10th Air Force, Captain Linden Johnson was busy in his tent, planning dive-bombing missions and reconnaissance flights and coordinating agent drops in the heart of the enemy jungle. When Lamont and Eldon walked in on Linden, maps spread out before him on his desk, he looked up. Astonished, Linden jumped to his feet and the three brothers just stood there for a moment, speechless. This was the first time that they had been reunited since they had entered the service several years earlier.

Amazingly, they could not have chosen a better day for their reunion, as Myitkyina was captured by U.S. and Chinese troops. However, as the brothers toured the area in a jeep and noted the death and destruction around them, they realized how blessed they were to have found each other alive and well. Later that day in a promotion ceremony, Lamont pinned to Linden's collar the gold oak leaf clusters of a major. Newly promoted Major Linden was granted relief from duty the next day to accompany his brothers back to Assam where, after a final night together of laughter and memories of childhood and home, Lamont bid farewell and returned to Karachi and his reprovisioned liberty ship. The threesome would not see each other again until after the war, in Kansas, eight thousand miles from Myitkyina. Though they cherish the memory of that muddy, monsoon-drenched, jungle meeting, to a man they are in agreement that there's no place like home.

•••

BIOGRAPHY: *Eldon "Johnny" Johnson was born in 1921 in Wichita, Kansas. His enlistment in the U.S. Army Air Force took him to India and Burma, where he piloted the P-47 Thunderbolt in the 10th Air Force and gained the final rank of major. As a civilian, he just couldn't get away from airplanes, working in upper management at Boeing. Now retired, Johnson "can be found piloting his powerboat over the waters of the Pacific Northwest."*

Reindeer Flight

—— By Commander Whit Johnson, USN (ret.) ——

as told to Milo James

In 1961, I was assigned to Fleet Tactical Support Squadron Twenty-Four Detachment, or VR-24 Det., the "World's Biggest Little Airline." Our mission was not glamorous in any Hollywood sense of the word, but during my tenure we played a role vital to the readiness and morale of the Sixth Fleet. One of VR-24's mission-critical functions included delivering cargo, personnel, and, perhaps most importantly, mail to aircraft carriers cruising the waters of the Mediterranean.

Regardless of how well equipped and trained a nation's naval forces may be, nothing rises to the same level of importance to sailors at sea, away from family, friends, and those cultural icons that anchor a man to the land he calls home, as the mail. This fundamental principle is in effect with particular poignancy during the holidays, when a longing to be with loved ones—trimming trees and covertly wrapping presents behind closed doors—infuses the long, hard days aboard ship with a bittersweet reminiscence. In mid-December, therefore, when my plane, a Grumman C-1A Trader (bureau number 146048), was due for overhaul and repair (O&R), the officer in charge (OIC) approached me and my crew with an idea.

The OIC suggested that my plane's final mission—a three-segment, five-day transport flight—before its scheduled O&R be flown, not by Lieutenant Commander Whit Johnston, copilot, and crew, but by a seasonally uniformed Santa Claus skipper and crew of Uncle Sam's top elfin aviators. Our maintenance team dutifully and merrily rose to the Yuletide challenge; 146048 emerged from several hours of unscheduled, unofficial holiday overhaul a forty-two-foot long, piston-engined, twin-prop, U.S. government–owned sleigh.

The first leg of this festive flight, dubbed the "Reindeer Flight," began in Naples early one morning and ended in Naples the afternoon of the following day. We landed in Barcelona and Rota, Spain, on the first day, and in San Javier and Palma Majorca, Spain, before returning to Capodichino Airport the second day. In each instance, local civilian dignitaries and senior military officers met the Reindeer Flight, exchanging smiles or salutes with the suspiciously svelte (but appropriately jolly) naval aviator and his crew, while clusters of junior officers and enlisted personnel cheered in childlike anticipation of the arrival of letters and presents from home. Word of our special mission preceded our arrival on the mission's third leg in Sicily, Malta, and Athens, where we met equally gracious fanfare.

Unlike Reindeer Flight's first and third segments, which included ground landings only, the second leg brought holiday cheer to the sailors aboard the USS *Shangri-La*, a Ticonderoga-class attack carrier then in her third month of a seven-month-long Mediterranean cruise. Our flight plan for that Wednesday—"Naples direct to CVA-38 and return"—would involve landing somewhere in the Mediterranean on the *Shangri-La*. Stretching some 888 feet from bow to stern, the 150,000 shaft horsepower, four-screw *Shangri-La*, rising nearly 100 feet above the sea and displacing over 27,000 tons of water, was a veritable floating city.

This buoyant borough, home to a crew of more than 3,400 men, brought with it everything necessary. Aboard her were probably 300,000 ballpoint pens, 1 million sheets of paper, and 80,000 rolls of toilet paper. The galley would certainly prepare as many as 11,000 meals each day, while in any given twenty-four hour period the crew would doubtlessly consume upward of 100 dozen eggs, 400 gallons of milk, and 450 fresh-baked loaves of bread. Sick bay would likely receive 6,000 patients in a year, and the barber shop cut over 150 heads a day. For all its preparedness, however, the one missing element aboard the ironically named *Shangri-La* was family. Mail from home, then, was a poor, but critical, surrogate.

This in mind, after our briefing, we made for our plane under dawn's early light. Against the boisterous, serious backdrop of NAF Naples, we presented a comically surreal dichotomy in our red and green "uniforms" while we strode purposefully across the tar-filled, grease-stained tarmac. The temperate breeze kept catching my faux beard, tickling my face as it danced upward. Clambering aboard the plane, despite our unorthodox appearance, we professionally completed our preflight checklist.

Taxiing to the runway's end and receiving clearance from "North Pole control" for takeoff, I advanced my C-1A's throttle. The twin 1,525 horsepower engines roared; cylinders firing, the nine-piston engines drove the huge propellers (with a torque efficiency that Dasher, Dancer, et al. would have envied) that grabbed the air, pulling the plane ever faster down the runway. Reaching takeoff speed, we lifted from the runway with an ease that contradicted the aircraft's somewhat whale-shaped profile.

Leaving behind the Bay of Naples, the romantic islands of Capri and Ischia, and nearby Mount Vesuvius, I brought my plane on course over the Mediterranean. The panorama from my windscreen was dazzling; shimmering thousands of feet below, the opalescent sea glistened in the morning sun, sharply defining the picturesque Italian coast. After an hour or so, when I was about seventy-five miles closing on the *Shangri-La*, I radioed in. "This is Reindeer Flight inbound on your one-eight-zero degree, radial seven-five miles."

"Roger, Reindeer Flight. Continue inbound. Signal Charlie," the radio crackled, giving me the go-ahead to begin landing ops. "Fox corpen two-four-zero degrees," the LSO continued, noting—by the etymologically enigmatic term—the ship's magnetic course heading for landing.

I began going through my landing checklist. I "dirtied" my C-1A, lowering landing gear, flaps, and tailhook—the hydraulic steel hook vital to bringing the 20,000-plus pound C-1A to a dead stop in seconds by catching one of four arresting cables on the carrier's flight deck.

The carrier in sight, I continued my straight-in approach toward the *Shangri-La*'s landing strip, which was angled about eleven degrees port of the ship's bow-to-stern axis. Of course, unlike rooftops on which Santa is accustomed to landing, this landing strip was attached to a ship, which, because of the landing strip's angle, was steaming not only forward but also away from any aircraft trying to land on it. So, I had to "crab" Santa's sleigh—flying both forward and sideways—lest the landing area slip away at the intended moment of touchdown.

In the groove, I saw the Fresnel Lens—a round light left of the ship's stern, which, when appearing amber to the pilot, indicates a properly angled descent—and called the meatball.

"Roger, ball. Looking good," the LSO responded.

I adjusted my angle of attack and continued to "fly the ball" in, keeping it even with the row of green horizontal lights on either side to ensure my plane's proper attitude, controlled my speed, and maintained my angle of descent. My copilot acknowledged, "Landing checklist complete," but then on final approach noticed I'd neglected to open my emergency escape hatch.

When I reached up and opened the hatch, a rush of air came into the cockpit, and my beard flipped up, covering my face. Not being able to see, with absurd futility I blew—*"phhhhh"*—and then desperately tore off the beard. Not a moment too soon. My peripheral vision immediately caught the relative (and damn fast!) upward movement of the ship's bridge toward my right; nanoseconds later my tailhook caught the number-three wire. In moments and meters, the cable brought my aircraft to a jolting stop.

I taxied up the flight deck, folded the plane's wings, cut the engines, and replaced my beard. The crew opened the main hatch and I climbed down. With Santa carrying a full mail bag and his crew carrying presents, the ship's CO, officers, and men greeted us. Stopping momentarily for the requisite photo op, we headed below deck. From the briefing room, we went to the galley for a quick lunch—something more substantive than a plate of cookies and milk, as I recall—and then reboarded our sleigh.

Taking off, the powerful *whoosh* of the flight deck's catapult propelled us to the *Shangri-La*'s precipitous edge and out over the deep, rolling sea. After a brief drop immediately after clearing the flight deck, Santa and crew soared upward. We left the ship and her crew behind, grateful not only for another safe landing, but also for that magically subtle joy that graces the heart on giving a gift whose value is not measured in dollars and cents. Here, the gift was hearth and home, wrapped in familiar handwriting and smiling photographs, in scented letters, in the innocent irony of a child's present purchased with mom's and dad's money, in the praise of a proud but worried parent, in the hand-scrawled anecdotes of old friends.

Of course, I could not help thinking, as we roared out of sight, "Merry Christmas to all, and to all a good night!"

•••

BIOGRAPHY: *Whit Johnson grew up in Connecticut along the Long Island Sound and early in life fell prey to the lure of sailing, flying, and snow skiing. Whit attended the University of Pennsylvania until, during the Korean War, he joined the Navy. Some twenty-two years later, Whit retired and began a new career in real estate. Single throughout his Navy career, Whit married Carol, an artist, when he was forty-nine years old. Today, the Johnsons enjoy traveling and sailing out of the balmy waters of Pensacola Bay, Florida.*

Fuel-Cell Failure

By Commander Susan Kilrain, USN

STS-83 launched on April 4, 1997, my first space flight. Seated in the cockpit in my orange launch-and-entry spacesuit and glossy black visored helmet, I focused on my responsibilities as *Columbia*'s pilot. Just after 2:20 in the afternoon, the solid rocket boosters (SRBs) ignited and *Columbia*, shaking violently, lifted off the pad. The engines roared deafeningly, and outside, the launch area—aglow with the orange-white-hot incandescence of burning fuel—filled with billowing blue, white, and gray smoke. Looking straight up, back to the ground, I saw nothing but the clear sky into which I was propelled.

About two minutes after liftoff, the SRBs separated from the shuttle's large, orange external tank, and continued their own ascent briefly before falling to be recovered in the ocean below. After another six minutes, the main engines cut off, and a few seconds later *Columbia* jettisoned the external tank, which disintegrated as it reentered the atmosphere, its pieces splashing into the sea sixty miles below. Traveling eastward after liftoff—at a speed increasing by two thousand miles per hour every minute—day soon morphed to night, azure to violet, and stars suddenly appeared amidst the inky blackness surrounding me. I was now in space.

The first day of the sixteen-day mission progressed smoothly, if busily, while I tried to adapt to space. However, on day two, Mission Control reported that, because of a malfunction with one of our fuel cells, we might have to shut it down and return early. On day three, Mission Control did order us to shut down the fuel cell and prepare to return to Earth next morning. I should not have been surprised; you see, I am a Navy test pilot. I've trained to fly many different Navy aircraft. My first A-6 Intruder flight—cut short due to a hydraulic system failure—required an arrested landing at Naval Air Station (NAS) Oceana in Virginia Beach. My first EA-6A Electric Intruder flight—cut short due to an engine failure and subsequent hydraulic failure—also required an arrested landing, this time in Key West. And on my first F-14 Tomcat flight, high oil temperature in one engine required an engine shutdown; unable to get the hydraulic crossover or restart the engine, I was forced once again to take an arrested landing at NAS Oceana. The only surprise, then, when my first shuttle flight ended prematurely should have been that a hydraulic system wasn't directly involved.

Actually, I was a little surprised; no mission had been cut short like this before. The engineers on the ground had always determined the cause of any problem, always found a way to safely continue despite any anomaly. This time, however, there was an indication a fuel cell was not working properly. If the signature—the data communicated to Mission Control from *Columbia*—was accurate, the fuel cell could start a fire, one of the two most feared emergencies in space (loss of cabin pressure being the other). Three fuel cells, by a reaction of liquid hydrogen and oxygen, produce all the electricity aboard the shuttle and, as a by-product, drinking water. With one fuel cell down, we could safely remain in orbit using the remaining two cells. However, this required reducing the electrical load significantly, turning off all nonessential equipment. This included the cabin fan—which functioned as a sort of air purifier—so that all the dust, lint, and other floating air particles now found their way into our eyes, mouth, nose, and lungs. Of course, the principal problem was that if a second fuel cell failed, we could no longer safely continue; de-orbit and landing require too much electricity. Technically, it's possible, but everything must go perfectly.

The world had had high expectations for us—sixteen days of combustion and material science on the first Microgravity Science Laboratory mission. Now, however, we were unable to deliver. Feelings among the crew were mixed; while disappointed, we also felt glad to do what safety required. Still, there was a small ray of hope—management sent a note a short time later, hinting we might refly the mission. I think most of us assumed they were just trying to cheer us up. It worked; vivified, we discussed how great it would be to fly again, to complete the mission, but did not really believe it would happen. You can't just schedule a shuttle flight anytime you want. But, it was fun to dream about flying again.

Meanwhile, a lot went through my mind. As the pilot, the fuel cells were solely my responsibility. The fuel cell switches are oddly positioned in the cockpit, situated vertically number-one over number-three over number-two, rather than number-one over number-two over number-three. Training, of course, stresses not shutting down the wrong fuel cell, so this was my primary concern. I also thought about the many scientists who'd been patiently waiting a very long time for their research to be completed on this flight. And, I reflected on my own disappointment, much like a child's on receiving only one gift at Christmas, wonderful though it may be, when expecting another, even greater present. We had just begun orbiting Earth on my first trip into space, and I was just getting my "space legs." Yet, I hadn't even had time to look out the window at Earth or take any pictures to record the biggest event in my life. But, I felt disappointment certainly less poignantly than others. Our commander, Colonel Jim Halsell (USAF), didn't want to go down in history as the only commander to cut a trip short. And our payload specialists, Drs. Roger Crouch and Greg Linteris—specifically chosen for this flight because of their scientific expertise—knew this was their once-in-a-lifetime space flight.

In any case, we had about thirty-six hours to take care of the fuel cell, complete as much science as possible, and prepare for the return home. Most of the time, we kept lights off to conserve electricity, using flashlights for illumination—holding them in our mouths when necessary as we worked—while performing our tasks in zero gravity, surrounded by the hum and whir of computers and other machines, and hundreds of displays and controls.

Occasionally, I'd take a little break and peak out the window. My initial impression on seeing Earth from space for the first time was that it appeared much closer than I'd expected. Unlike in photographs first taken by the *Apollo* from the moon, I could not see the entire planet. Instead, our altitude—184 miles—presented a vista more similar to that from an airplane, though the curvature of the earth was much more well pronounced. It was, nonetheless, awe inspiring. The shuttle orbits "beneath" the planet (for various reasons, the shuttle is upside-down relative to the earth, so the earth appeared to be above the shuttle) every ninety minutes at about 17,500 miles per hour, resulting in a spectacular sunset or sunrise every forty-five minutes. Each sunrise illuminated cottony clouds floating over the planet's tan, brown, and brick deserts and plains, and blue and green oceans, rivers, jungles, and forests; and each sunset awakened millions of tiny city lights in the darkness of the earth's populated areas and billions of stars visible from the other side of the shuttle.

Once the specialists had deactivated the lab, we turned the lights on, spent some time filming, and then, on our sixty-third trip around the globe, prepared for de-orbit and landing. Reentering the atmosphere was a bumpy ride and generated what felt like tremendous G-forces but was, in fact, less than even one G. Outside, there was a vibrant glow of fiery red, orange, yellow, and white streaks. By eighty-three thousand feet above the earth, we'd slowed to two and a half times the speed of sound. At ten thousand feet, having already rumbled through the sound barrier, we were now less than a minute from touchdown, gliding quietly—the shuttle, having no power of its own, is effectively a one hundred–ton glider—toward the runway only a few miles ahead. At three hundred feet, I lowered the landing gear and, *Columbia* alighting gracefully onto the runway, deployed our red-white-and-blue drag chute.

After landing, we exited the shuttle. In the crew quarters, I was elated to see my husband (then, boyfriend) and my father, whom I hugged, smiling. After we got out of our space suits, we met with the chief of flight crew operations, who told us management was serious about reflying the mission. If it could be worked out, we would fly as early as July. We were overjoyed at the possibility, but cautious, not really believing it would happen. A few weeks later, though, management determined that our mission's importance required a second flight. Only three months after STS-83 landed, we launched again as STS-94, conducting, this time, one hundred percent of the planned science experiments, and completing both the full sixteen days ... and my second trip to space.

•••

BIOGRAPHY: *Susan L. (Still) Kilrain was born on October 24, 1961, in Augusta, Georgia. She always dreamed of becoming an astronaut. Now a veteran of two space flights, Kilrain has logged over 471 hours in space on two shuttle missions. Married to Navy SEAL Colin Kilrain, she's the mother of two. Commander Kilrain is currently assigned to the Office of Legislative Affairs at NASA Headquarters, Washington, D.C.*

Images of War

By Joseph Kraynak

as told to Milo James

When the Japanese attacked Pearl Harbor, I was already a sergeant, having enlisted in the Army in 1940 and been promoted on an accelerated basis. Notwithstanding my infantry training, the Army offered me the chance, which I accepted, to join an artillery air-observation section, whose mission was flying light planes over enemy lines to direct and adjust artillery fire on enemy targets. After air observation school, where I became intimately familiar with the Piper Cub—a two-man, fabric-covered monoplane that I could dismantle, load onto a truck, and, in less than two hours, reassemble—I transferred to Headquarters Battery, 29th Field Artillery Battalion, 4th Infantry Division.

In January 1944, we shipped out to Axminster, a small town in Devon County, England, to continue training for Operation Overlord, the invasion of Normandy. On June 4, though, a gloomy, wet day, I had to leave my unit—and the friends with whom I'd trained and worked and bonded—for Southampton, England, at a time when everyone felt a very potent sense of an impending "something." Thoroughly dejected, when I arrived at Southampton I could not believe what I saw there. Moving about in the rain in a flurry of activity were columns and columns of soldiers amassed with myriad artillery pieces, mortars, tractors, trailers, half-tracks, jeeps, and all sorts of other weaponry, equipment, and vehicles.

Next night, we moved out. After boarding an LST (Landing Ship, Tank)—a 380-foot-long amphibious troop and vehicle transport ship—we steamed out into the murky English Channel. I felt a little scared, of course, but did not know what exactly to fear. Lying uncomfortably in the dark among the trucks, tanks, Higgins boats, and other GIs, my fear grew, becoming as palpable as the damp air. At dawn, despite the low fog, the veil of night lifted, exposing thousands of boats and ships as far as the eye could see. Suddenly, filled with a contagious confidence, we at once began cheering, some even daring to venture, "This is gonna be a piece of cake!" and wondering, "How can anyone stop us?"

At about 0900 hours—I went ashore in the third wave, the first having landed in the dark about two or three hours earlier—we began transferring to the Higgins boats, the high-sided amphibious-assault boats with the drop-down steel door at the bow, for transport to the beach. Confidence waning, just as I thought, "This is gonna be bad!" it got worse. Instead of boarding a Higgins boat, I had to join my disassembled airplane aboard a Rhino Raft, a flat, seventy-foot-long, motorized raft of conjoined, steel-pontoon sections that offered zero cover from enemy fire. Fortunately, though, there was little German opposition then, save for some attacks from the pillboxes on the shore. Reaching shallow water, we drove onto the wet sand of Utah Beach, and immediately the grim reality of war became clear as guys from the first wave returned, wounded or dead, for transport back to England.

By now, the fog had burned away, and it was becoming a beautiful, warm day. Our first objective was to meet up with the 82nd Airborne—which had parachuted in behind enemy lines in the middle of the night—and liberate the little town of Sainte-Mère-Église. My immediate task, though, was finding a football-field-sized clearing in which to assemble my plane and from which our pilots could take off to fly missions.

Conceptually, our missions were simple. We'd fly ahead of our positions, about one or two hundred yards from the German front line at altitudes from five hundred to one thousand feet, which was pretty scary since, although the lower we flew the better we did our job, we also became better targets. When the Germans first saw our diminutive Piper Cubs flying low overhead, they paid little attention (they just assumed we were dumb, I think). However, after noticing a correlation between our presence and the accuracy of our artillery salvos, we started taking small-arms fire, and lost a number of planes and pilots that way.) Our mission responsibilities did not include calling in grid coordinates, knowing specific targets, or even initiating contact with our command post (CP). Instead, we'd know in advance the general area of our CP's intended targets and, after spotting their first few rounds, conversationally radio in adjustments: "too far," "too short by one hundred meters," etc. In this way, we primitively but very effectively walked in the M-101A1 Howitzer rounds until right on top of the target. At that point we'd give the go-ahead, "FIRE FOR EFFECT!" and up to four batteries would bomb the hell out of the gun emplacement, truck convoy, ammunition dump, train, or whatever the target happened to be. From our bird's-eye view, we could see and hear the *VAROOM* of the explosions—orange and white and black, just like in the movies—the rounds often flying pretty close to us because of our position.

The images of the invasion were ghastly. It felt so unreal, surreal; I could not believe I was there. As we marched toward Sainte-Mère-Église, disheveled and scared, the day grew hotter and the smell of death hung offensively throughout the area. By noon, dead livestock— victims also of explosions, bullets, and shrapnel—punctuated the countryside, bloated to grotesque proportions under the midday sun. I saw downed Allied gliders, smashed up either from having been shot down or merely from rough landings. I saw paratroopers suspended in trees by the lines of their parachutes, shot dead by the Nazis—surely one of the most pitiful things I've ever seen in my life. One particularly poignant incident was an epiphany for me, however. I'd come across a dead German, his weapons still on him. Taking his rifle and Luger pistol, I searched him and, finding a worn leather wallet, took it from his wool uniform. Discovering inside a family photograph, I stood over his lifeless form, realizing my enemies were no different from me; we were all just a bunch of kids following orders. I could no longer hate them. Duty and honor, of course, not to mention the need to keep myself and my buddies alive, required me to keep fighting. But inside, the misplaced hatred evaporated.

As we fought our way across the hedgerowed Norman farmland—the small fields were separated by mounded rows of earth, trees, and shrubs in which the Germans would sit in wait—I was struck by the presence of countless Polish, Czech, Russian, and other Slavic refugees the Nazis had conscripted into slave labor. Though liberated by the Allied push across Europe, they were still homeless, country-less, hungry, and poor, separated from family, either by death or distance. Sometime after we retook Cherbourg but before liberating Paris, I met two sad, suffering Russian boys—Nikolai and Stefan, about thirteen or fourteen years old—among the refugees, and my heart just went out to them. I fed them some of our wax-packaged rations, which, though pretty crappy tasting, were good food. They liked us so much they kept following us. So, I "adopted" them. They stayed with me for some nine months, helping me with my mundane tasks, the three of us somehow communicating. I tried to get permission to get them back to the States, but failed, and, after a time, we just had to let them go. Sadly, we lost touch after separating; I truly wish we had not.

The war, as brutal and gruesome as it was, offered some moments of levity, born of the bond unique to comrades-in-arms, that, without a doubt, helped me get through it all. Especially memorable are the time I "liberated" a half-dozen cases of cognac from an MP-guarded barn—filled floor-to-ceiling with wooden casks of France's best brandy—in the middle of a farm (I thereafter became the de facto package store for my battery), and the time we finally met up with the Russian Army south of Berlin. By then, there was no way the Nazis could stop us. In this momentary union of East and West, we had a wonderful time; happy to see each other, we hugged and endeared our-selves to one another in vodka and smiles, each of us recognizing a *tovarish* in the other.

Shortly after meeting the Russians, I went home. Leaving behind a ravaged continent and not a few dead friends, I've kept with me all these years the memories, the good and the bad, which, together with the friendship of great men with whom I proudly served, have helped make me the very grateful husband, father, grandfather, and American that I am today.

•••

BIOGRAPHY: *Joseph Kraynak was born in 1921 in Weatherly, Pennsylvania, the son of Pennsylvania coal miners. In 1940, Joe enlisted in the Army. After World War II, Joe returned to Pennsylvania, where he met and married Stella. Still married after nearly fifty-seven years, Joe and Stella have eight children and thirty-one grandchildren. After completing his GED, Joe attended art school in Pittsburgh and became a commercial/industrial artist. Now retired, Joe continues to paint and restore art.*

Sailors' Currency

By Petty Officer First Class
David K. Kresge, USNR

In the fall of 1986, I was a Petty Officer Second Class assigned to VP-11 at NAS Brunswick in Brunswick, Maine. VP-11 (the Pegasus) flew the Lockheed P-3C Orion, a land-based, four-engine, turboprop aircraft whose primary mission was conducting antisubmarine warfare (ASW) and maritime surveillance operations in opposition to the Soviet naval threat. Because of the logistical, tactical, and strategic importance of the waters surrounding Greenland, Iceland, and the United Kingdom, we frequently flew missions out of and trained in the United Kingdom, often jointly with the British.

Participating that fall in a six-week exercise with the Brits, VP-11 flew out of Royal Air Force (RAF) Base Machrihanish, in Machrihanish, Scotland, a picturesque little village on the Atlantic coast of the Kintyre Peninsula. The exercise pitted the Brits and Americans as opposing forces, one blue, the other orange, battling in simulated combat. So, when those of us in sub hunters were flying missions, we'd utilize our infrared, acoustic, and magnetic detection devices to locate, track, and "kill" one another's submarines.

Off duty, we competed on a bit more friendly level, though no less earnestly. One evening in a local pub, while hoisting a few pints and talking sports with some of our newfound RAF friends, one of my fellow squadron members, Jack, had engaged a Brit in some good-natured, competitive "trash talking." Jack accused the Brits of being soft—"wimps" was what Jack called them, among some other, more salty words—for playing soccer rather than American-style football, and the Brit gave it right back. Their bantering drew the rest of us into their tête-à-tête, and before long, the Brits challenged us to a game of American football, with a wager attached, of course.

After flying the following morning's missions, we all gathered for the match-up—Uncle Sam versus Her Majesty—at a large field at RAF Machrihanish with thick, soft, natural turf for our gridiron. It was a perfect, football-fall afternoon, sunny, temperature in the mid-sixties with a slight chill in the air. Everything was intensely green and the landscape beautiful, just like in pictures or movie scenes of Scotland—rolling hills as far as the eye could see and tons of grass and clean, fresh air, the ocean visible in the distance. We marked off the field the same way we did as kids playing in the street or park, delineating out-of-bounds with an imaginary line between two trees on one side and a tree and a fence post on the other side, and the end zone similarly.

My team had dressed for the game in shorts and T-shirts, so the warmth of the sun felt pleasant in the chilly air while we waited for the Brits to show up. When they did arrive, they struck me as rather comical; while they'd challenged us to a game of our own co-national pastime, they were the ones dressed for the part. At least some of them, anyway. A handful of the Brits wore cleats, one had on football pants, another arrived with an American-football helmet, and one guy even wore shoulder pads.

Each team fielded a regulation, eleven-man squad. As the two teams lined up for kickoff, the "fans" on the sidelines—local Scots, and Americans and RAF guys who did not play—cheered their respective teams, clapping, encouraging, and jeering. The game went back and forth, and at halftime we led. On defense, I played defensive back and, together with our other DB, both of us fast, slightly built, and wiry, showed the Brits the value of a furious and frequent blitz strategy, chalking up tackle after tackle.

Each side played for keeps. There were some shoving matches, and toward the end of the game, when we were down one touchdown, our injury roster listed three men: one with a broken collarbone, another who'd hyperextended an arm, and a third with a sprained ankle. Still, we had possession and were driving downfield—until, that is, a lieutenant from my squadron showed up. Seeing in our football match only the destruction of Navy property (namely, us), he ended the match then and there, which is one of the reasons we lost (that, and the sun got in our eyes). The lieutenant was, apparently, unimpressed with our method of establishing good international relations but, though he gave us a pretty good talking-to, no one got in big trouble, which was fortunate given the injuries we'd sustained. Bottom line, though, we lost.

Fully chagrined, covered with dirt, and with grass stuck to our clothing, sweaty skin, and matted hair, we went to the barracks to shower and change. Once cleaned up, I headed off-base with a large group of my teammates not scheduled to fly the next day—it being verboten to drink within twelve hours of flying—and took taxis into Campbeltown, a charming Scottish fishing village, with narrow streets running between well-kept Victorian row-homes and corner pubs. Climbing into our hackney, I told the driver to take us to Splash!, a local public house where we were to pay our debt to the victors in the sailors' currency of lager and ale. During the ride, the driver asked whether we were part of the group that had played football that afternoon. We said yes, and then he, laughing at us, gave us a hard time because we'd lost at our own sport. If the cab driver knew of our ignominious defeat, the whole town would know!

Our several cabs arrived at the same time. Paying our drivers, we entered the crowded, dark pub, heads held high. It was kind of like Norm entering Cheers. As portended by my cabby's ear for gossip, most of the patrons had heard the story before we arrived and, of course, also razzed us mercilessly. Joining the RAF guys at the bar, we opened a tab and made good on our wager. Throughout the night, we played darts, hoisted pints of Tennent's lager, and sipped tumblers of Springbank single malt in a haze of cigar smoke—forced, as I recall, to toast the Queen, the RAF, and the British Empire.

That football game was more than a game. It further established, albeit slightly, the ties between the guardians of freedom of the two greatest nations on Earth. Moments of levity like that between allied troops contributed to winning the greater "game," the Cold War, because without the cooperation and high morale of the NATO nations, especially the United States and the United Kingdom, the world would no doubt be a frighteningly different place today. "Cheers" to my old friends from RAF Machrihanish. We did good.

• • •

BIOGRAPHY: *David Keith Kresge was born in 1965 in Lansdale, Pennsylvania. He enlisted in the Navy in 1984, serving four years' active duty. A lifelong resident of the greater Philadelphia area, David graduated from Temple University in 1992 and began a career in technology. Employed as the computer/network systems administrator for a large health-care management provider, David continues to serve in the Navy Reserves.*

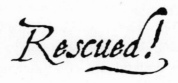

Rescued!

By Wilson F. Leon

as told to Milo James

Fifteen thousand feet over the Mediterranean, I sat on three flak suits in the top turret of a B-24 Liberator, manning a Browning .50-caliber machine gun. One of seven bombers tasked with blowing up a rail yard in Salonika, Greece, we left Naples, Italy, at just past 0500 on September 24, 1944, an absolutely beautiful Sunday. From my lonesome perch, around me I could see the other planes in formation over the sea below.

Not far from our target, we began taking flak from antiaircraft guns below. The first four rounds missed, leaving puffs of black smoke in the air. The fifth round, though, hit the plane in front of mine, right in the center of its fuselage. The B-24 exploded, disintegrating in a humongous ball of yellow flame that we flew right into, rocking my plane and taking out the entire formation. Of the seventy men aboard the seven planes, only eleven survived.

As we passed through the explosion, I rushed down to the flight deck and looked around. The pilot was gone, and the copilot, and the bombardier, the navigator, nose gunner, radio operator, everyone. Even "Peanuts," our five-foot-five crewman who manned the ball-turret, another machine-gun-armed Plexiglas globe suspended from the plane's underside. I grabbed the last parachute from the flight deck, put it on, and jumped through the open bomb-bay doors, dropping into the cold slipstream. When I released the parachute, it opened forcefully, and the poorly fitted harness pulled hard on parts of me better left unpulled. Wincing, I looked down and watched my plane dive toward the ground. I never saw it hit, though; my attention had turned to the Germans driving along a highway toward a lake where it looked like I would land. Suddenly, I heard sounds coming from my parachute canopy and thought at first that birds were flying into my parachute, until I realized the Germans were shooting at me.

When I finally hit the ground—faster than I'd expected, so I tumbled backward pretty hard and bruised a leg and rib—I stood up immediately and saw my enemy driving toward me, now about fifty yards away, shooting at me. Since there was nothing I could do and no point in running, I dropped and waited.

They took all eleven survivors prisoner, marching us through the streets of Salonika to the airport. Ten of us came from my plane. The eleventh was badly wounded, his arms burned, the flesh hanging grotesquely from his limbs. As we walked through Salonika, I noticed my leg was bloody, that I'd taken a bullet or piece of shrapnel from the explosion (I don't know which since it went clean through). Trying to remain in good spirits, I pointed out to my buddy, Homer, the cute Greek girls along the street, until a guard shut us up. A little Greek boy—the cutest kid you ever saw—threw a pack of cigarettes at me; I later used the cardboard from the box to secretly keep a mini-journal during my captivity.

When the Germans first interrogated me, they brought me to a large, empty room. There, a long-haired corporal and a high-ranking officer stood, waiting. When the corporal, translating for the officer, asked me my unit and similar questions, I answered with name, rank, and serial number. But, when he asked how many men were on the planes they shot down, like a dumb son of a bitch, I answered, "Well, tell me how many men you have and I'll tell you how many men were on the planes." His jaw dropped. The officer spoke sharply to the corporal and the corporal turned and replied, and I thought I was dead where I stood. But they didn't kill me. They didn't even hit me (they'd taken care of that previously, actually). They just let it go for some reason.

Though they originally intended to transport us out of there by plane, at about 1700 hours a few American planes strafed the airfield and shot up everything. So, they took us to the roundhouse at the rail yard—the one we'd intended to bomb—to board a train. When we left Naples that morning, the weather was perfect, so when they captured us, we were in shirtsleeves, pants, and boots; no more. When I saw an old rain coat, then, half-buried in grease and gunk on the roundhouse floor, and knowing that winter was near (and the mountains nearer still) I pulled it out, shook it off, and brought it along.

They put us in one end of a boxcar, all eleven of us plus a Russian pilot with a bad leg wound. On the other end, some German soldiers and naval officers lounged in relative comfort. As the train pulled away, heading toward Yugoslavia, the Russian pilot, writhing in agony, began calling out over and again for water. The Germans, eating and drinking water from their canteens, ignored him.

The train made several stops that day. At the first stop, they took the crying Russian away, and he never got on again. At another stop, I watched between the slats of the boxcar as a second train pulled alongside us. An SS trooper jumped off and, approaching our boxcar, opened the door and looked in. When we first got on the train, I'd wanted to stay by the door, figuring if anything happened, I could get out of there first. So, when the SS trooper looked in, he saw me and took me and Homer off the train and made us give him our boots, lest we attempt an escape. We followed him to a gondola car where he ordered us to unload it. Barefoot and gloveless in the snow and freezing rain, we unloaded all of its scrap-metal cargo for what seemed like hours.

When we'd finished, the SS soldier refused to return our boots. Fortunately, however, a higher-ranking Luftwaffe officer saw him and ordered the soldier to return our boots; clearly, there was a hierarchy of humanity among our enemy. In fact, somewhere on this trip, I ran into the officer who'd interrogated me at Salonika. When he recognized me, he stopped me. Struggling with heavily accented English, he said, "You know, Sergeant, vee should geef Roose-felt a gun und Hitler a gun und let zem shoot each other und vee can get zee hell home."

Life in the train soon became pitiful. We did what we could to stay warm; Peanuts used the filthy rain coat I'd taken from the round-house as a blanket. If we had to urinate, we'd just roll over, piss in the straw, and hope that it would drain away from us. Before long, the rancid stench from our buddy's burn wounds began seeping through his masking-tape-like bandages. For several days we traveled like this. After dark, we tried the best we could to sleep. Late on October 4, however, a tremendous explosion rocked the train. The Greek partisans had blown up the tracks, taking out the train's engine and the first four cars. I don't know how many died or were wounded, but after the confusion, the Germans unloaded their horses and wagons from the train, and we marched to a prison in Skopje.

Next day, we set out again, marching on foot behind the horses. At night we'd stop near streams and they'd let one of us get a bucket of water, but still did not feed us. Peanuts was always right behind me, following me because I was older; he was a tough kid, but still young and, like the rest of us, scared. We continued like this until October 18, when we arrived in Mitrovitsa where they imprisoned us in a makeshift camp with what must have been several hundred other prisoners.

My weight when we left Naples in September was about 180 pounds. When we arrived at Mitrovitsa, I weighed about 120 pounds, and Mitrovitsa didn't help. Our quarters were foul and grim, boasting a couple of straw mattresses on slats. I lifted my mattress and looked; scurrying about, if there was one bloodsucking bedbug, there were five hundred. So, during the day we'd just sit outside in shirtsleeves, huddled together with our backs against the shed, killing lice between our fingernails. I could feel them crawling over me; their bites festered badly because the Germans did not feed us, not anything worth calling food, anyway. Every day we each had a small loaf of bread and a cup of bean soup. The bread was about as big as half a canta-loupe until we cut off the green mold, leaving not much more than a golf-ball-sized meal. The soup was black on top from the bugs that come out of the beans when cooking, but we'd scrape off the bugs, eat the residue, and then get sick as hell.

We left Mitrovitsa for Novi Pazar on November 5 and spent the next couple of nights in the woods without incident. On November 7, we stopped for the night in the hilly woods far from any town. Suddenly, an accented voice hollered out of the darkness, "Run Americans! Run!" From out of the darkness they materialized— Chetniks. They were everywhere, rifles trained on our guards. The Germans' dogs were barking. Several rifle shots rang out, followed by a sharp yelp or two that quickly faded. One Chetnik walked up to one of our guards and laid into him with his rifle, delivering a powerful butt stroke to his mouth, then, grabbing him, cut his throat and announced, "We don't waste bullets." While all this transpired, of course, we scrambled to get the hell out of there.

The Chetniks didn't let us run far on our own, thankfully. The next several weeks we stayed at farms where they treated us well until a Bulgarian soldier came along and we left with him. After several days following railroad tracks and hitching rides on Bulgarian Army trucks, we reached a camp about thirty kilometers from Sofia. After days of red tape (some things military are universal), we went to an American mission in Sofia, and from there flew to our old outfit in Naples. Finally, aboard the USS *West Point*, we steamed through the Mediterranean and zigzagged across the ocean to Boston. And, cold as Boston was, I was damn glad to be home.

•••

BIOGRAPHY: *Born in 1920 and raised in western Pennsylvania, Wilson Leon worked for a trucking firm and on the docks in Pittsburgh before enlisting in the Army for World War II. After the war, during which he was awarded the Purple Heart, Leon went into the moving and storage business, where he rose through the ranks to head his company. Retired almost twenty years, Leon and his wife reside in Jacksonville, Florida.*

Every One, Precious

BY SANFORD "SANDY" LEBMAN

as told to a friend

A reporter from my hometown paper in Ventura, California, once asked me whether I hate the German people. In the beginning, of course, I did. Witnessing what happened to my father, to my family and our heritage, left me very embittered. After I arrived in Europe during World War II, got into battle, and began taking prisoners, the other guys in my unit would use my hatred as a psychological weapon. Since I was the only Jew in my unit, the other soldiers would bring the German prisoners to me and, gesturing toward me, would say, "Jude" (pronounced "yú-de," German for "Jew"). That was all it took; the German prisoners would turn ashen, wide-eyed in terror. The other guys always felt that as long as our prisoners knew I was Jewish, they'd not give us any trouble. It was true. The prisoners were afraid of me. I mean, they were really afraid of me. They could see it in my eyes that I could just as soon kill them as not.

But, my hatred did not last forever. After two particular incidents with German locals, where I learned the Germans could love as well as hate, I no longer had it in me to hate, either. Assigned to an armored cavalry unit, my job was to run reconnaissance patrols behind enemy lines. One time, on a foot patrol with nine other men about ten miles behind enemy lines, the Germans had just made a successful counter-attack, cutting us off, and we desperately had to find cover. Finding a farmhouse, we entered, prepared to kill everyone inside so we could hide. We asked the German family living there whether there were any German soldiers around. They said no, but that the Germans were coming this way. Amazingly, though we treated them quite roughly at first, they took us in, hid us from the German soldiers, and—perhaps because I was the youngest—treated me like a son. The walls of the rooms in their home were lined with deep drawers. So, while the rest hid in the barn, three of us hid in these drawers, the family letting us know when it was safe to come out to go to the bathroom and to eat. (Once, I remained in a drawer for three days!) We remained there—this family, whose name I never learned, feeding us, protecting us from the German soldiers, treating me like family—until, after an American attack, it was safe for us to leave.

Another family also saved us, this time from the elements. An elderly couple (with whom I just fell in love), Herr and Frau Haff lived in the Alpine foothills of the German-Austrian border. I met them toward the end of the war while in command of a small unit. Having determined that my men and I would use their home for shelter, I told the couple I would take their bedroom. This notwithstanding, the Haffs treated us so nicely I still can't get over it. One particularly cold night while I was asleep, my gun under my pillow—we could not afford to trust anyone—I awoke with a start when someone entered my bedroom. Grabbing my gun, I raised and directed it toward the sound, index finger pressing against the trigger, not quite heavily enough to shoot. I yelled out, "*Wer ist da?*"—German for "who is there?" It was Frau Haff, who'd come in to bring me an extra blanket. "Oh, God," I thought. "I almost killed her!"

While these encounters with German locals defused my hatred, its heinous source was beyond words. And I saw it, firsthand. In April 1945, I was out in front of enemy lines again, in Bavaria, on reconnaissance near the town of Dachau when I first saw the camp. Initially, I did not know it was a concentration camp; I thought it was a prisoner-of-war camp. Spotting a guard, I got out of my armored car to get a better look at what exactly was in front of us. Suddenly, guards began shooting at me, so I ran back and jumped in my vehicle and told my driver to crash the gate. With three of us in the first armored car, my driver sped through the gates, the locks giving way to the weight and force of our vehicle. Once inside, what I saw. . . .

Stacks of dead, naked bodies littered the grounds. Mounds of them. Heaps of corpses everywhere. (I still can't cope with having seen the railcars stacked with bodies, overflowing with death.) Against this surreal, Dante-esque backdrop, we fought the guards, ferociously, inside the concentration camp. And though I had to radio for the infantry to come help us out, of course in the end we won. Decisively. Looking around at the silent horror, I thought, "I wonder if any of these are my dad's relatives. My relatives." They could have been, of course. I just don't know.

In spite of the countless dead, many did survive. Not just Jews, either, though most were; also interned there were educators, doctors, anybody who disagreed with the Nazi regime. Regardless of who they were, though, they happily greeted us, "Comrade, Comrade!" The historical question of whether the Allies should have bombed the concentration camps is to me a question that implicates not just the sanctity of life, but of lives. For though I do not pretend to know whether it would have been better to bomb the camps, I do know this: Each one of the survivors I met after liberating Dachau is precious.

●●●

BIOGRAPHY: *Sanford "Sandy" Lebman was born March 13, 1925, in East Liverpool, Ohio. Lebman enlisted in the Army as a private and left as a Second Lieutenant. Married fifty-eight years, Sandy and his wife, Lois, are proud of their four children, four grandchildren, and two great-grandchildren. They live in southern California.*

Setting Sun

By Milton Lisansky, D.D.S.

as told to Milo James

After receiving my D.D.S. from NYU and completing basic training in 1943, I began active duty in the Army Dental Corps, practicing routine dentistry in various locations in the United States. In autumn 1944, the Army assigned me to the 88th Field Hospital at Camp Ellis, Illinois. A newly activated unit, we spent several months preparing for deployment and, in early 1945, sailed from Fort Lewis, Washington, to Hawaii for jungle training and amphibious landing operations in preparation for—though we did not know it then—Operation Iceberg, the invasion of Okinawa.

In late March 1945, I left Honolulu knowing only that I was headed for a combat zone. Steaming westward across the Pacific, we stopped at several islands, including the tiny volcanic atoll of Ulithi (home to the then-largest and most covert naval facility in the world). In late April we pulled into a harbor in southern Okinawa and anchored amidst thousands of ships; as far as the eye could see, navy-gray- and "dazzle-camouflage"-painted ships sat anchored in the blue waters.

My APA's cranes lowered into the water the Higgins boats—boxy, thirty-six-foot wooden amphibious assault boats—used to ferry troops and supplies to the beach. I climbed the rope netting hanging from the ship into one of them. We landed on Higashi Beach, where a month before the Tenth Army had landed relatively unopposed.

While we waited a couple of days for our equipment and vehicles to be ferried in from the APAs, I witnessed for the first time the horror of a kamikaze attack. High in the sky—at first it was no more than a black dot against the blue sky—we spotted a single Japanese bomber circling. At once, thousands of ships opened fire, the kamikaze their sole target. Above the harbor's calm surface, the reports of the vessels' antiaircraft guns thundered and filled the sky with bright flashes and black smoke. Every ship was firing when the kamikaze suddenly turned and dove. Despite the tremendous firepower unleashed against him, the pilot crashed his plane directly into the USS *Birmingham* (CL-62). The impact of the suicide plane's five-hundred-pound bomb ripped through three decks, including its sick bay, killing forty-five. Instantly, all guns went silent. As the reverberations of the explosion faded, a smoke ring rose over the 610-foot cruiser's fiery deck. Watching in shock, we all said the smoke was the soul of the pilot.

Not long after, all our matériel had been transported from the ships and we turned our attention to setting up our field hospital. With as many as three hundred beds, our site quickly became a small city of olive-drab tents, jeeps, and ambulances splashed with the familiar red cross on a white background. Within a few days, American casualties began arriving. A twenty-four/seven operation, we functioned as the first instance of definitive care, other than that provided at field aid stations. Against the background sounds of artillery, in the feverishly paced operating room, I participated—with the guidance of surgeons, of course—in tasks for which dental school had not prepared me.

This went on until the last week of June, when the Japanese on Okinawa began surrendering in large numbers. Almost immediately, American casualties stopped arriving. Under new mission parameters, we converted our site to a POW hospital, increasing to twelve hundred the number of beds and adding a barbed-wire perimeter and armed guards. On the eve of receiving our first Japanese wounded, the officers held a meeting. There, we discussed whether we'd give penicillin (which was not available to the American public) and whole blood to the Japanese rather than sulfur drugs and plasma. We decided we had to go with the plasma and sulfur drugs, reserving the penicillin and whole blood for Americans. Once we began treating the prisoners, however, we used the blood and antibiotics as we would have for any other patient, and that decision was never again discussed.

After a time, the stream of casualties decreased and things calmed down—for the most part. During the Japanese suit for peace after we dropped the twenty-two-kiloton Fat Man atomic bomb on Nagasaki, the rumor mill churned. One night, every antiaircraft (AA) battery on the island started firing, illuminating the dark sky with search lights, explosions, and luminescent trajectories. This was unusual; normally the AA guns fired in a linear progression, one battery firing first, then, stopping, its searchlights would go out and the next battery would open fire. While the aircraft were not visible, we could track them by the correlative progression of AA fire. So, since we could neither see nor hear airplanes on this night, and since every AA battery on the island was firing, the rumor—and consequent fear—spread of a tremendous counteroffensive of black-clad, black-parachuted Japanese paratroopers invisibly dropping out of the night sky. Far from the case, however, the guns had unleashed a volley of celebratory salvos as a rumor of Japan's official surrender went around; ironically, the "friendly" fire that night wounded many Americans.

After the war, I managed to arrange a transfer to Kure, Japan, where I served as the medical officer of an ordinance battalion. I remained in Japan during the occupation for nine months. I took great interest in fraternizing with and learning from my new Japanese acquaintances, and fondly remember that time. When I finally went home, I was able to bring with me—in addition to Japanese weapons, Kodachromes, and memories of war—memories of friends I'd made and the cultural education I'd received during the occupation.

...

BIOGRAPHY: *Milton Lisansky, D.D.S., was born in 1918 in New York City. In May 1943, Lisansky reported for active duty in the U.S. Army's Dental Corps. Honorably discharged from the Army in September 1946, Dr. Lisansky was in private dental practice until his retirement in 1982. An accomplished amateur photographer, Dr. Lisansky enjoys music and theater with his wife, Sybil.*

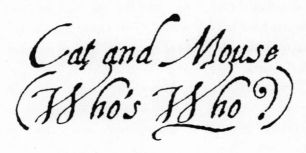

Cat and Mouse
(Who's Who?)

By Anonymous
as told to Morgan Lo Re

I guess there are many stories and stories within stories. Perhaps one might say that within these stories there are truths within truths. Vietnam had three stories. The government's story, the story that the press told, and the story as lived by those who served.

One of the stories that the public was told stated that there were no Americans in Cambodia. And why should there be? Even though there were an approximated twenty-five thousand North Vietnamese troops in Cambodia, it seemed that the *New York Times* thought Americans should not be in a neutral country. I imagine "Nathaniel Victor" (North Vietnamese Army) was "invisible," and the Hanoi press reports were the standard by which the *New York Times* writers wrote their stories.

So with this in mind, I found myself "somewhere" in Cambodia. It wasn't the first time, and it wasn't going to be my last time given the fact that I wasn't "really" there and the NVA (North Vietnamese Army) weren't "really" there either. This being the case, I guess no one actually existed out there at that time. My unit didn't truly matter since it *didn't exist.*

125

But Cambodia existed and so did the heat, the tall grass, the thick jungle, the insects, the adrenaline, and the fear. Now a soldier does not like to use the word *fear.* He would much rather think that he is, shall we say, alert. Given that we were always in "Indian country," we were always VERY alert!

Our mission was to locate enemy troops, avoid contact if possible, and report back. Since we knew who we were, anyone else we ran into had to be the bad guys. We knew we were the good guys because "God was on our side." (Where have I heard that before?)

Well some strange things can happen as they can happen only in combat. There were eleven of us as I recall, and we had been in the bush for two days. Two days in Indian country can make you a bit edgy, and we were edgy. So far, we had observed no enemy forces, and it appeared that Mr. Nathaniel Victor was not home. Perhaps he had gone on vacation. But as luck would have it, in the fading light, visibility became even more difficult and a strange thing happened. [The two "nonexistent" parties] walked smack into each other. Funny how the vanishing light and thick foliage can make something like that happen.

No one was really sure if they actually got a good look. It was more of a movement—sound—stop movement—reaction kind of thing. It happens fast, but it is always in slow motion. It was too late. Both sides knew the other was there though we were all well concealed.

We operated when possible with hand signals as per past missions, training, et cetera. But most importantly, we anticipated each other's reactions as only a small unit can. I signaled up three fingers and pointed, counted off three with my left hand, and four of us started to "rock and roll." This means that you are on full automatic, and as soon as you go through a clip you reverse it. Then you slam in the other clip, which is taped to the original clip.

While we rocked, our people spread out for two reasons. One, we were going to try to sucker Nathaniel Victor into a kill zone. Our second reason was to make sure that our "friends" did not outflank us. But a funny thing happened. Instead of getting full blasts back from our "friends," we heard only three or four AK-47s barking back. The other funny thing was that they started rocking and rolling at the same instant we did. I had this feeling that there were more than three or four of them out there. You see, in any of the recon (reconnaissance) work I had done, I had never seen or heard of only three or four NVA. There were always more of them grouped together.

The problem was, nobody really saw anybody; we were laying down fire into the bush and so were they. Now everyone was moving low but not slow. We opened the door for them, but they would not walk in, and they opened the door for us, and we would not walk in. It seemed no one wanted to go to dinner. How many were out there? What had we run into? I am convinced my counterpart was thinking exactly the same thing.

Well, after a couple of minutes we took more fire. The fire wasn't from the same position, and I knew the original shooters had not moved that far. Now I knew for sure there were more out there trying to "channel" our movements. Of course, we returned some fire, but it was not from our original shooters. I was trying to "channel" them. Both of us were playing cat and mouse, trying to coax the other side to commit. But who was the cat and who was the mouse? My North Vietnamese friend and I were mirroring each other's thoughts and tactics.

It being the first date with my counterpart, I was not ready for a lifelong commitment. He, no doubt, felt the same. It was time to end the date and try for true romance another time.

After some defensive maneuvering, we took off. In other words, we "beat feet," "got out of Dodge," "diddie moue." It might seem funny, two groups of soldiers running into each other, both sides unloading and then getting the hell out in the opposite directions, but that's the way the day went down. Personally I missed the humor in the situation.

Not much of a story, you might think. No great heroics. Not even a Band-Aid on our side.

In my debrief, I told my story, said I thought there were more of them than us and that they were trying to suck us in. I went over my tactics, which were recorded for future reference. I explained how my opposite mirrored my strategy. My guy looked at me and said, "Okay, good job. We have some other reports. Sounds like you ran into some lead elements of at least a regiment. Get your people some rest; you're going out again in two or three days." Case closed.

The way I see it, we made contact and brought back our intel. Other reports helped firm up the picture. We had a substantial NVA troop concentration on the map! No doubt in my mind, in a very short time, some "fast movers" that did not exist would be swooping in and dropping nonexistent "snake and nape" (bombs) on some nonexistent North Vietnamese troops in a part of the war that never happened.

But the real story here is that all my people made it home.

• • •

BIOGRAPHY: *This Special Operations specialist was born in New Jersey. As a child, he grew up "with his boys," playing football and causing mischief. After college, he was recruited for Vietnam in Special Operations where most of his duty occurred in Cambodia. After serving, he began a career in technology. Married, he has three children and lives in northern California.*

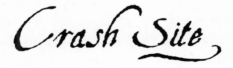

Crash Site

BY STEVE LUND

23 April 1969—one of those inky black nights that often occur in the tropics where the sky is overcast and there are no city lights illuminating the landscape, the darkness seeming to envelop us like a black velvet curtain. I was working on top of the engine deck of a helicopter, a UH-I Huey, with a crew making rigging adjustments to the fuel control. We hoped to complete the work so I could test fly the aircraft at dawn the following morning. Turning to the team chief to say something, I heard the whine of a turbine engine close by, followed by the muffled sound of an explosion coming from behind the buildings to the rear of our hangar. I looked past the chief in the direction of the noise and saw flames erupt over the top of one of the low buildings that bordered the road to the rear of the complex.

For some reason, I did not immediately connect the sound of the engine and the flames with the crash of an aircraft. Instead, because of the explosion and flames that continued to leap above the level of the buildings and hangar, I thought an enemy rocket round had landed in the hospital complex—a fairly common occurrence at Cu Chi at that time—and had set a building or something else on fire. I jumped down from the Huey's engine deck, shouted to the maintenance team leader to call the base camp fire department for help, and ran toward the flames.

When I rounded the corner of the tech supply building, an image for which I was totally unprepared confronted me. It wasn't a burning building at all; it was a burning helicopter. One hundred feet in front of me, in the middle of the road, was a U.S. Navy UH-IE Huey completely engulfed in flames. As I ran toward the aircraft, a man emerged from the Huey's cabin and was running toward me. Two others then cleared the cabin, leapt a ditch behind the first soldier, and moved forward. To my sudden horror, I realized that they were on fire.

As I approached the two burning men, Burt, a Specialist Fourth Class, ran past me with a small fire extinguisher in his hands. Together, we met the desperate men, colliding with them. Burt sprayed them both with the fire extinguisher at point-blank range. His prompt action undoubtedly saved their lives, as their clothes were fuel soaked and we could never have put out the flames in time to save them by rolling them on the ground and beating the flames with our hands, as I had initially intended to do.

As I got up and continued toward the aircraft, I could see the pilot struggling to free himself. His leg appeared to be trapped. The flames inched toward him as Burt and I leapt the ditch just thirty feet away, when the fuel tank exploded. The explosion hurled us both back as if one giant fist had struck us with an outrageous force. To this day, I pray to God that in that moment of explosion the pilot immediately died without suffering, because when I looked up after regaining myself from the blast, he was slumped over, completely engulfed in flames. As I watched, the form that only seconds before was a full-sized man, burned down to a residual lump no larger than a wastebasket. Never in my life have I seen a more horrible sight, and I could do absolutely nothing to save him.

As I watched the pilot's death, I became aware that the hair on my arms, with which I shielded my face, was quickly burning away. I rolled, trying to escape the heat and the flying debris and shrapnel that were landing dangerously all around me. But then I saw Burt lying unconscious about ten feet away, shirtless as our enlisted men often were when working in the torrid jungle. With the heat from the fire intensifying exponentially, I realized our own peril. Crawling over to Burt, I shielded his body with mine.

I was wearing a Nomex flight suit and thought it could protect us both, though it certainly would have been more effective had I thought to roll down my sleeves. I still carry the scars from that mistake as a reminder. But the most vivid images and "scars" occurred in the following few minutes after I wrapped my body around his—and those images are forever etched eerily in my mind:

My face inches from Burt's, not knowing if he was even alive.

Something hitting me in the back like I had been kicked. (I still have the object that hit me, a spent .50 caliber shell casing I retrieved the next day.)

A basketball-sized sphere of metal, glowing cherry-red, landing two feet from my head and bouncing off into the darkness.

Numerous small projectiles hitting my back and legs, and constant dread that the next would be bigger.

The sudden realization that Burt's eyes were open.

A lull in the din, scrambling to my feet, and pulling him along with me.

We half-ran-half-dragged ourselves to a nearby fence. My pant leg caught in the barbed wire and ripped as I pulled it free. Hands from the other side of the fence, grasping at us from out of the darkness beyond the fire, pulled us to safety. The darkness was alive with moving people all around me, but I could not see them. I lost contact with Burt; no matter, he was in safe hands, secure from the terrible heat and the flames that had seemed to be reaching out for us.

I turned around and looked back toward the burning Huey. The blazing aircraft cast a bright pool of light, making the darkness around us all the more intense. I was alone, surrounded by faceless people, chaos infusing the night. As the flames began to die down, the cockpit became recognizable.

Then, the awful, heart-rending reality that the small, burning black lump in the flames was a man—whom I tried to the utmost of my ability to save but failed—began to creep over me. In utter misery, I turned away, unable to bear looking at it any longer. I wandered to the other side of the tech supply building. The quiet, inviting darkness beckoned me. I was filled with an overwhelming and desperate need to be alone. The resolve that sustained me through the last half hour was slowly slipping from my grasp. I have never known such a feeling of complete defeat in my entire life. I was beaten. I could have been that man's salvation, and I had failed. He had died horribly, watching his unsuccessful would-be rescuers as they sought to reach him.

My calf brushed against the low sandbag revetment that surrounded the building, and, sitting down on it, I buried my face in my hands and did something I hadn't done since I was a child. I began to weep.

Sometimes one's life reaches such an ebb that one can go no lower, can feel no greater suffering; I had reached that point. All the pain of that night and strains and hardships of the previous months in Vietnam burst forth in tears. It was as though a floodgate had been opened and the wretchedness of all the previous defeats of my life had spilled out.

I don't know how long I sat there that way, unnoticed and anonymous in the darkness. It doesn't really matter. When I got up, the feeling had begun to subside. Things were starting to come back into focus. It would be days before I began to see it all in perspective; some aspects of it would take years. But, for now, I was numb. The body adapts; that's why we experience shock. I only discovered my physical injuries—the burns on my arms—when back in my hut while sitting on my bed in a reasonably composed state.

I had indeed failed to save the life of the trapped pilot, and the man who had truly saved the lives of the two burning crewmen was Burt—though others said Burt would have died where he had fallen if I had not shielded him and dragged him to safety. I don't know. Only God knows. With a single explosion, He had decided everything. Had it happened a few seconds earlier, we would have still been out of harm's way. Had it been a few seconds later, there would have been three burning lumps in the inferno.

•••

BIOGRAPHY: *Steve Lund was born in Bagley, Minnesota, in 1947 and raised in Washington and Oregon. Lund departed for Vietnam in December 1968. He transferred to the Army Reserves in 1975, from which he retired as a lieutenant colonel in 1995. As a civilian, Lund worked in the aerospace industry as a commercial helicopter pilot and Chief of Human Factors Engineering for Hughes Helicopters. He's currently a pilot for the California Department of Justice.*

Too Close for Comfort

—— By Lieutenant Colonel John H. Matthews, USA (ret.) ——
as told to Milo James

Hue/Phu Bai, Republic of Vietnam, 1968. It was a pleasant late-spring day, clear, not too warm, and relatively dry. I'd just ducked out of my battalion's bustling operations center after a morning of briefings, situation reports, and mission plans to take advantage of the weather. To the west under the blue sky sat a range of lush, rolling, grass-covered mountains.

As the operations officer for 1st Battalion (Airborne), 321st Field Artillery supporting the 101st Airborne Division, I'd been serving in our tactical operations center as the fire direction officer after arriving in-country only a few months ago. Ever since moving into LZ Sally, just north of Hue, we'd been taking mortar, rocket, and small-arms fire nearly every night. Sometimes during the day, too. My duties, of course, included trying to locate the shooters and forward observers that had to have been encamped somewhere in the mountains. Raising my binoculars to scan the ridgeline, I searched for any signs of the enemy. Suddenly, I spotted movement along the ridge.

Immediately calling for our pilot, he and I jumped into our battalion's H-23 Raven and took off, flying toward the mountains. From the open-sided "goldfish" bubble of our chopper—similar in

appearance to the H-13 Sioux familiar to fans of the TV show
M*A*S*H—I spotted more enemy movement on top of the mountain.
In the din of the whirling rotor blades, I called in the grid coordinates
to two of our M-102 howitzer batteries. In minutes, the mountainside
erupted in a furious barrage. A dozen-plus high-explosive 105mm
shells, some timed for airburst and some for point detonation, whis-
tled through the air and slammed the ground. Orange-and-black fire-
balls blasted the earth, *KABOOM,* hailing shrapnel, dirt, flora, and rock
fragments amidst the surreally idyllic surroundings. In spite of the
105's three-hundred-meter casualty radius, it was obvious that the
howitzer shells' trajectory was too low, rendering the salvo ineffective.

Grabbing the radio again, I called 1st Battalion, 377th Field
Artillery (one of the first ARA designated battalions in Vietnam),
which supported the 101st. In short order, a platoon of two UH-1B
Huey helicopters—equipped with two side-mounted, 2.75-inch
rocket launchers—joined us. The sky filled with the *whuup-whuup-
whuuping* of rotor blades and, under my fire direction, the Hueys flew
several sorties, unleashing burst after burst from their twenty-four-
round rocket pods. Flying low over the enemy emplacement, the Huey
pilots reported no movement and several bodies.

In artillery, we didn't often get to confirm the effectiveness of an
attack, since those who survived dragged away the dead and secured
any remaining weapons and intelligence before we could get our assets
to the target area. But this time, the Hueys, circling protectively above
anyone who might have lived through that high-tech inferno, were
ready to unleash a flurry of 7.62mm rounds from each of the Hueys'
two pintle-mounted machine guns if necessary. So, after convincing
my pilot I needed to go in, I radioed Battalion HQ for permission.

As we descended, I counted the bodies on the ground. Twelve.
Tightening my steel pot's chinstrap, I jumped out just as the landing
skids touched ground on the far side of the mountain, the tall grass
dancing wildly from the whirlwind under the chopper's blades.
We'd landed about three-fourths of the way between the crest and a
foxhole about forty meters below the ridgeline. Pulling my sidearm—

an M-1911A1 .45 caliber pistol—from the holster snug against my olive drab fatigues, I shouted to the pilot to keep the chopper running and got a thumbs-up in reply. One of the Hueys circled overhead, while the second landed on the ridgeline uphill to my right.

Quickly and carefully, I headed toward a group of figures sprawled, dead, in the grass beyond the foxhole and its ominously silent occupants. Reaching the bodies, I was surprised; they were not Vietcong, as I'd expected, but North Vietnamese Army regulars—the VC's more well-equipped, well-trained, and well-disciplined benefactors. I glanced around carefully and picked up a Soviet AK-47 and some SKS Chinese carbines, and then checked the bodies for documents. Grimacing, I caught a whiff of some seriously rank nuoc mam, the salty, high-protein fish sauce the Vietnamese ate with nearly everything. Slinging the rifles over my shoulder, I darted uphill and, ducking under the spinning blades, loaded them in my chopper and headed for the foxhole.

It must have been balefully obvious how easy and attractive a target I was at this point, tall (even in a crouch) in the afternoon sun, the guy responsible for making this a very bad day for these North Vietnamese. Lowering myself into the foxhole, I was met again with the pungent odor of nuoc mam. I retrieved rifles from the dank floor and moved the corpses, searching the foxhole for documents, and made a mental note of the current body count—nine. Gathering notebooks and other papers, I clambered out of the foxhole, looked around, and returned to the chopper.

"One more time!" I yelled to the pilot, and headed back downhill, mindful that my current body count was three short of the twelve I'd spotted earlier. After a final search of the foxhole, I climbed out and turned to look downhill. Suddenly, from behind me there erupted the terrifyingly unmistakable *KRACK-KRACK-KRACK-KRACK-KRACK* of automatic weapons fire, and I heard an inner voice declare, "I'm going to die!" Expecting the inevitable—bullets crashing into my body—I whirled around toward the source. Still unscathed, however, I saw that one of our door gunners had fiercely but purposefully opened fire from the crest. A dashed, phosphorescent path lit up the air about four feet above the ground, tracers flying downhill. Before I could spin further, the bullets found their target. In fractions of a second, multiple rounds had traversed a deadly course from the Huey, thudding into the torso of an already wounded North Vietnamese soldier behind me. I reeled around in time to witness a now lifeless form—lifted off the ground by the impact of the rounds hitting him at nearly twenty-eight hundred feet per second—crumple to the soft earth, still holding a rifle in one hand. He was not even ten meters from me.

Running to him, I grabbed his weapon, dashed to my chopper, and scrambled aboard. "Let's go! Let's go! Let's go!" I yelled, animatedly pumping a fist, thumb upturned. Getting the hell out of there, I radioed over to the Huey's pilot and told him to pass on my most sincere thanks to his door gunner, who had just saved my life. Looking down as we sped away, I counted again. Ten bodies. Three of us were very lucky indeed, that day.

••

BIOGRAPHY: *John Matthews was born in Laurel, Mississippi, in 1939. He served in the U.S. Army from 1961 to 1983, including four years as an assistant professor of mathematics at the United States Military Academy at West Point (USMA). After retiring from the Army, Matthews worked for GTE and Rockwell, and served as vice president and general manager of Mason and Hanger National. He and his wife, Nancy, parents to three and grandparents to seven, live in Pensacola, Florida.*

Nameless Few

By Chaplain (CAPT) Robert McMeekin, USAR

On the evening of September 10, 2001, while preparing to seal an opening in a closet at home, it occurred to me that my family should enclose a time capsule in the wall. So, my wife, my children, and I each placed in a box items that best illustrated our faith, lives, and hopes for the future. Next morning, our world changed forever.

There was no question among my friends in the military after the terrorist attacks that we'd go to Afghanistan if called, though I'd dismissed my own chances, as my last deployment had been less than eighteen months earlier. Several months passed. Sunday morning, January 27, began normally. I'd just donned my black cassock and pectoral cross, preparing to leave my house for Liturgy, when the phone rang. "Chaplain," the voice from the 644th Area Support Group at Fort Snelling, Minnesota, said, "you need to get down here immediately. You're to report for duty in Afghanistan in seventy-two hours."

Less than three weeks later, my assistant, Noah, and I arrived in Bagram, Afghanistan, in the dead of night after a four-hour flight from Turkey. The plane landed in total darkness—no lights inside or out. One of the ground crew drove us to the ATOC (Air Transportation Operations Center) to log in and wait until morning to find our point

138

of contact. At 0630 hours, when the snow-white mountains around us began slowly to materialize out of the waning darkness, we met with the 10th Mountain Division chaplain in a large, bombed-out hangar, after which he ordered us to find a place to bunk down and sleep for a few hours.

In my nearly nine years as an Army Reserve chaplain, I never expected to see a combat zone. Yet, here I was. When I arrived, Operation Anaconda, the allied attack on an al Qaeda/Taliban stronghold in the Sha-I-Kot Mountains, was less than two weeks away. In that time, Noah and I learned quickly, readying ourselves to respond without hesitation when casualties and fatalities arrived. On the eve of Anaconda—which would involve the fiercest fighting in the war to date—Noah and I familiarized ourselves with the Mortuary Affairs facility.

That evening, our soldiers prayed, ate, and bedded down early before moving out in the middle of the night. Following stirring speeches by our commander and sergeant major at a rally, the Protestant and Catholic soldiers filed off to their respective corners to receive Holy Communion, while I—there being no Eastern Orthodox soldiers present—made myself available to all others, including, despite the Cross on my cap, reciting the She'ma and Sabbath Prayer in Hebrew with three Jewish soldiers.

Next morning, at daybreak, we received news that one Special Forces soldier, CWO Stanley Harriman, had died. Soon, American and allied Afghani wounded began arriving in waves. So much happened that long first day and night. Heavy mortar fire had pinned down elements of the 1st Battalion, 87th Infantry Regiment, killing CWO Harriman and wounding twenty-six. Others, whom machine-gun fire had pinned down for over sixteen hours, arrived both hurting and very cold from their prolonged exposure to the frigid mountain air. Chaplains and assistants scrambled to help any way we could. In the hot, frenzied emergency room, doctors and nurses cleaned wounds and extracted shrapnel and bullets from torn body parts.

Lengthy periods of waiting and praying punctuated the intervals between arrivals of wounded. With one dying Afghani soldier, I prayed

"God is Great!" four times and the prayer of repentance in English. A nearby medic, hearing me, queried, "Do you think he understands you?" "In death, all is understood," I snapped back—surprising myself—and the medic nodded. Another soldier with whom I prayed, Kyle, had lost a toe. After praying, I asked whether I could do anything for him. When Kyle, his expression serious, apologized for answering yes, I thought, "Ah, a profound theological question!" Then he asked, "Father, do I qualify for disability?" (Oh, my arrogant presumption!)

After the initial shock, we counted the wounded, comparing names and social security numbers. I'd now been awake for nearly twenty-two hours. Before going to bed, I stopped by an ambulance to pray by CWO Harriman's remains. Laid out on a litter, his head rested in a crimson puddle from a gunshot wound. As a parent, I imagined the young man as a child, his mother cradling him and his father patting his head and tousling his hair. As I prayed, I thought of his family going about their daily tasks back home, dreaming about their son, praying for his safe return. Knowing that in less than twenty-four hours a drab-colored government car would pull up to their home, its somber, uniformed occupants bearing the tragic news, I prayed for them, also.

During that long ordeal, I prayed with most of the wounded that came to us, as did the rest of our chaplains. Evident, as I watched my colleagues, was the love they had for these guys, and the humility I'd been feeling in the presence of these heroes commingled with pride and a sense of privilege at working with such fine chaplains. The war also afforded the chance to serve with ministry teams from our coalition partners, some of the finest chaplains in the world. I served with chaplains from the Polish engineers and the Royal Marines, and chaplains from various German, Italian, and Dutch units. That Easter, many faithful gathered on the airfield ramp-way for an ecumenical sunrise service, at which the Royal Marine chaplain played "Amazing Grace" on the bagpipes, with A-10 Warthog ground-attack airplanes loudly taking off in the background. Later that day, British and American soldiers gathered together at a memorial service offered for the Queen Mum, who'd passed away the day before—on Holy

Saturday, the day Christians lament the buried Christ while simultane-ously anticipating dawn to celebrate His Resurrection.

During my tour, my division chaplain, ministry team, and the coalition chaplains were exemplary. We can achieve much more than the emptiness of ecumenical luncheons and tiresome utopian speeches; we can become a living faith committed in love to a living people. Loving God as He loves us and encouraging and leading others to love Him, though simple, is so overlooked in the world of spires, domes, cassocks, and collars; we religious types fuss over so many trivialities that we miss the very stuff of life. Fr. Alexander Schmemmann, of blessed memory, often wrote that what is lacking in the Church is simply living in the Kingdom of God. For me, it took a combat zone to pare away all the chaff I've held up as wheat. Perhaps few can say that the Army has made them better husbands, fathers, or priests, but I can; in this desolate place, all has become precious. The Army does not often build shrines to chaplains. No, if we nameless few have had any lasting effect, it's because we've left our soldiers with a newfound faith in and love for God. For if we are truly faithful and have found the wisdom to yield to God's sovereign agency, then we've learned the truth of salvation—that we "must decrease, so He can increase" (John 3:30).

•••

BIOGRAPHY: *Born in Brooklyn, New York, in 1960 and raised in nearby Yonkers, Fr. McMeekin received his undergraduate degree from the State University of New York, Geneseo, before graduating from Luther Seminary in St. Paul, Minnesota, with his Master's degree in Divinity. Having later converted to Eastern Orthodoxy, McMeekin was ordained an Orthodox priest after completing the Late Vocations Program of the Orthodox Church in America. An amateur paleontologist and student of numerous foreign languages, McMeekin's other interests include fishing and hunting, model railroading, and politics and world events. McMeekin and his wife, Julie, a registered nurse, parents to three children, currently reside in Wisconsin where McMeekin serves as parish priest to Holy Cross Mission in St. Croix Falls.*

The Jolly Green Giant

By "Miller"

as told to his daughter

When I was thirteen years old, my daddy went off to the war in Vietnam. Thirteen was an awkward, difficult year, and Vietnam was an awkward, difficult war. I survived my adolescence, as my daddy survived the war, but neither of us was ever the same again.

We never talked about it. Talking about it was something you just didn't do. Back then, the war was a taboo subject, in our house as in our country.

Twenty-two years later, I was asked to review a concert for the local paper. It was called "In Country" and it featured Vietnam veterans singing songs about the war. I invited the colonel to come along.

The guys in the band were great. The songs they sang were funny, painful, true—songs like "Danang Lullaby," "Freedom Bird," "The Ho Chi Minh Trail." But it was the song about the Jolly Green Giant that brought tears to my father's eyes.

The colonel is not the kind of guy who cries. I was stunned. After the concert, I took him to the nearest bar, ordered him a Chivas and water, and said, "Okay, Dad, tell me all about the Jolly Green Giant."

"Okay," he said, "but you can't tell your mother. Ever."

"Okay."

"It happened in Cambodia. The NVA had been stockpiling supplies about a mile across the border, and we seized them. The GIs were having a ball, trying on socks and riding bicycles and carrying on.

"The next day I took the general out for a look. We flew in on a Huey helicopter. Just as we approached the supply site, we were hit with 51-caliber machine-gun fire. They hit some hydraulic lines and the pilot lost control of the Huey. He did a steep turn and dive for the deck. It was a soft crash landing.

"The general was pissed. He kept hitting me over the head with his metal clipboard, screaming, 'You're trying to kill me, Miller, you're trying to kill me!'"

The colonel paused.

"Then what happened?"

Dad was reluctant to go on.

"Come on, Dad."

"We waited for the Jolly Green Giant."

I knew from the concert that Jolly Green Giants were rescue helicopters usually sent in to bring back downed pilots.

"You waited ... surrounded by fire?"

"Yep."

"What did you do?"

Dad looked at me. "I did my best to keep the general alive."

He didn't want to say any more, and he didn't have to. I'm a colonel's daughter; I can read between the lines.

"How long until the helicopter showed up?"

"About half an hour. That Jolly Green Giant was about the most beautiful thing I'd ever seen."

Dad finished his drink. I ordered him another one.

"The next day I got word that the general wanted to see me. I figured I was in some serious trouble for nearly getting him killed, and would be out on my ass by sundown."

"But when I got to his office, the general gave me a Bronze Star. Said, 'Thanks, Miller, for saving my life.'"

The colonel laughed. I raised my drink to him, and our glasses clinked. "That's a great story, Dad. Thanks for telling me."

"You're welcome," he said. "But don't tell your mother."

My mother still doesn't know.

•••

BIOGRAPHY: *"Miller" was born and raised in the Midwest. After joining ROTC in college, he was commissioned into the U.S. Army as a second lieutenant in 1954. He served his country for twenty years and retired at the rank of lieutenant colonel. I'm sure that he has lots more great stories to tell, but he's not talking.*

Nisei Legacy

By Hiro Nishimura

The story: My story actually begins fifty-five years after World War II, on June 21, 2000, at the White House ceremony celebrating twenty Nisei soldiers who received the Medal of Honor. The Department of the Army reviewed the cases of fifty-three Nisei Distinguished Service Cross (DSC) awardees for upgrade to Medal of Honor for wartime prejudice/discrimination prevailing during the war and in the military. After a year's review, twenty Nisei were recommended for the Medal of Honor and the awardees and/or their families were invited to the historical event. In the words of President Clinton about the honor, "It [was] long past time to break the silence about their courage. ... Rarely has a nation been so well-served by a people it has so ill-treated." One of the honorees was my friend Kazuo Otani.

Otani and I served together at Camp Carson, Colorado, for ten months in a segregated unit, performing the least-favored duties—duties like KP (Kitchen Patrol), guard, latrine, and rifle range. There, we bonded together under demoralizing discrimination, resigned to waiting out the war as second-class soldiers.

Our status worsened with the news of the uprooting of our families from the West Coast to internment camps in the desert areas. Our peers and brothers were no longer draft eligible. But just when all hopes were lost, news of an all-Nisei 442d combat team reached us and we were to serve as cadres. I remember Otani's jubilation. "Yeah!" he shouted, "we're going to be real soldiers now!"—and how true his words proved to be. Not only did the 100th Infantry Battalion/442d Regimental combat team see battle, but it also earned the distinction as the most decorated unit of World War II. The 442d boasts 21 Medals of Honor, 33 Distinguished Service Crosses, 559 Silver Stars, 4,000 Bronze Stars, and 9,486 Purple Hearts. Conservative estimates show that at full strength, the 442d numbered only 4,500 men—yet I've seen that the unit earned over 3,900 individual decorations.

Meanwhile, the Military Intelligence Service recruiters for linguists arrived. Because I so wanted to join the 442d with Otani, I planned ahead and stayed away from the barracks and the recruiters. I knew because of my expertise in Japanese and because I'd been studying at the university in the language, I'd be pulled for a linguistics area. But I got caught just as they were leaving the building. "One more," they said as I anguished over getting caught. Then, with forthrightness, I told the recruiters, "I'm not interested in studying. I wanted to go to Camp Shelby with my comrades." A terse "Okay" was my only answer, and they left. Honesty had worked; I considered myself a member of the 442d!

But then, without warning, a month later, I was taken in the middle of the night to Military Intelligence Service Language School. I was shipped out alone. I was upset and angry over my separation from Otani.

Soon, we lost contact as he went to Europe—and I, to India and Burma. While I interrogated Japanese POWs, somewhere my friend Otani was fighting bravely on the battlefields of Europe. After two years in the China-Burma-India theater, I happily returned home. But my joy was tempered at the news that Otani had lost his life, killed in action.

From that moment, Otani was on my mind. Where had he died? How had he died? Why did he have to die? I wondered about his family. How had they taken the news? Who would carry on his legacy? His story must be told. I searched for his kin. I looked for his hometown friends in Visalia, California. I even checked with "G" Company guys, but to avail; Otani's family, I learned, did not attend veterans or company reunions. I was frustrated; I had never been given the opportunity to say my good-bye to Otani. Time passed, and I was never able to find any news of Otani's last days. But again, Otani stayed in the recesses of my mind.

Then one day came the phenomenal news of the White House ceremony for twenty Nisei Medal of Honor awardees. How proud I felt as I started reading the names, and when Otani's name appeared, I just stared and kept staring. It was a very uplifting, emotional relief from my past frustration to see that he was being recognized for his patriotism and the sacrifices he made for this country. My relief, however, was temporary, as the old concern came back about his legacy, about his family carrying on his memory—an important aspect of our Japanese culture. Who was going to carry on his Medal of Honor legacy? Who would recall their ancestor, Otani, and his bravery in Pieve di S. Luce, Italy, July 15, 1944?

Meanwhile, the Japanese American communities everywhere were in a celebratory mood; both Los Angeles and Honolulu prepared for their memorial programs for the Medal of Honor awardees and their families. Excitement was in the air, and the media were everywhere. Then, followed the Seattle, Washington, memorial celebration for William K. Nakamura of Seattle and James Okubo of Bellingham, the two Washingtonian natives.

After the Seattle Medal of Honor program, a friend of mine, Tosh Okamoto, had an idea to implement a memorial dedication at Okubo's high school. Okamoto told me he had written to the city council and then to the mayor without a response for three months. I was moved by his desire for a dedication, and wrote to Mary Jane Kinoshita of Seattle, a friend living in Bellingham, for help to contact someone. She arranged a luncheon meeting with Jack Westford, son of the former city mayor, who offered his help in arranging the program. It was at this meeting that Okamoto mentioned James Okubo's brother-in-law, Clem Miyaya, living in Mercer Island, Washington. I told Okamoto that I was going to visit Miyaya to inform him of our plan. This turned out to be one of the most important decisions of my life.

As I had planned, I traveled to Miyaya's home—and it was there that I received my most memorable war story, a story not about me but about my friend, Kazuo Otani. After Miyaya and I talked about Okubo's high school plan, our conversation turned to the White House ceremony, and I learned he was there! I excitedly asked if Otani's kin were present. They had been! Moreover, Miyaya had given his kin a snapshot of Kazuo Otani. With this revelation, I was euphoric and ecstatic with relief and joy in finding my unexpected closure—finally.

When I explained my concern for Otani's kin, he startled me again by saying, "He was my sergeant. I saw him get hit!" I was shocked as he matter-of-factly shared the details of Otani's death. The platoon had become pinned down in a wheatfield by concentrated fire from enemy machine-gun and sniper positions. When one of his men was hit and left in full view of the enemy, Otani dashed out to his side to render aid. Quietly, I asked, "Was his demise quick?" Miyaya nodded, "Yes," as I sat fixated on the revelation of Otani's last moments. As I struggled to regain my composure, I sought comfort in Otani's heroism and honor.

As I recovered from the horrors of war implicit in Otani's death, my senses began to focus on my incredible good fortune on hearing Miyaya's revelation fifty-six years after the war. I wondered if it was due to a happenstance or Otani's legacy. I concluded it was neither one, as I realized that something so phenomenal must be both historically and culturally inspired. The Nikkei survival of discrimination and tribulation during the war years, the internment camps, and the post-war ostracism—all are a testament to fortitude and loyalty.

To share this story, I am grateful. I am most grateful to the legacy of all those Nisei soldiers who fought for the United States—proudly and bravely—thus opening the door to Miyaya's revelation and my surprising closure. I needed to know how my friend died and that his story would continue to be told, that generations would know the valor of Otani and that his family knew of his patriotism and strength.

•••

BIOGRAPHY: *Hiro Nishimura was born in Seattle, Washington, in 1919, as a second-generation Japanese American. He joined the Army in February 1942. Once discharged in 1945, he used his GI Bill at the University of Washington, and enjoyed a career in the university's Health Sciences department. He and his wife, Dorothy Hisako Yoshida, are the parents of three grown daughters, Celia, Robyn, and Karen. Now retired in Seattle, Nishimura is the author of* Trials and Triumphs of the Nikkei.

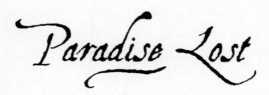

Paradise Lost

By "George"

as told to Allison Neyhart Rubin

I was on my second tour of Vietnam, and the Marines had just been positioned in a small town called Dong Ha, which is on the coast of South Vietnam near the border with North Vietnam. I was three hundred yards off a beautiful beach in a tropical area. The August air was hot and muggy, with temperatures in the 90s; rain showers fell often around that time of year. Any other time I would have loved to go there for a vacation. It was almost like a beautiful tropical beach in Hawaii—except that people were being killed.

At about 10:00 one morning, I got onto a hospital ship because we were expecting American casualties to arrive shortly. Soon, however, Vietnamese soldiers lined up on the beach and hid in palm trees; without provocation, they started firing small arms at our hospital ship. Although this was my second tour of Vietnam, and I was used to being attacked, I remained in fear of losing my life. Even though I was scared, my mission was to help our brave soldiers fight for the United States and return home safely. Staying focused on your mission can serve to keep your mind off the fear.

While standing on deck after the shooting from the palm trees subsided, I noticed a small Vietnamese canoelike vessel coming toward our ship. In it were two Vietnamese soldiers and a suspected Vietcong sympathizer whose hands were tied behind his back. When they were about two or three feet away, one of the Vietnamese soldiers put a gun to the sympathizer's head and killed him right in front of me. I heard a small bang, smelled gunpowder, and then felt blood splatter on my face. The top of the man's head was blown off, and there were pieces of human brain and skull everywhere, including on my uniform. Although I had worked in the hospitals and seen some grotesque casualties, this was the first time I had ever seen anyone killed directly in front of me. It hit home hard. Right before my eyes, I witnessed how quickly one person can take the life of another person.

Within split seconds of this shooting incident, a boat brought my best friend from the shore. He had stepped on a land mine. Both legs were gone, and he was losing large amounts of blood quickly. We took him to the operating room and worked madly to stop the bleeding. Because of my military training, I was able to divorce myself from any emotional thoughts; I needed to concentrate on the procedure. Unfortunately, we were not able to stop the bleeding, and he expired on the table. We soon found out that the land mine responsible for his death was one that the United States had given to the Vietnamese; then the Vietnamese had turned around and sold it to the Vietcong on the black market. Ironic, isn't it?

Those deaths were the most traumatic deaths I have ever seen. I've seen many people die: from old age, from car accidents, from knifings. Witnessing my best friend's death and seeing someone's execution are the most brutal memories I have ever had to deal with. After that, I realized that we were never going to win the war in Vietnam, and I felt sorrow for our young men who had to fight every day for a losing cause.

There is not a day that passes even now that war experiences don't filter into my thoughts. I feel compassion toward those who sacrificed their lives for the United States, and sympathetic for those who were affected by war in horrific ways. Whenever I visit Washington, D.C., I go to the Vietnam memorial wall and look up my deceased friend's name. The day of his death was one that is indelibly imprinted on every facet of who I am. Never do I want any of my children, grandchildren, or loved ones to ever be involved in war.

•••

BIOGRAPHY: *After serving as a medic in Vietnam, "George" returned home to his wife. They've been married for forty-three years and have three children and eight grandchildren. Now an oral surgeon, George hopes to retire soon and spend all his time playing golf.*

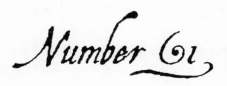

Number 61

By Jack Parks

as told to his granddaughter, Noelle Parks

One of my most memorable experiences about the Korean War actually took place while coming back from R&R (rest and relaxation). We'd just completed our time away from Korea in Tokyo, Japan. I remember looking around, my eyes squinting against the sun, and wiping my damp forehead with the back of my hand. About 250 young soldiers newly bathed and clean stood in fresh uniforms behind a crowded rope in an outdoor military airport in Tokyo. It was about 2:30 in the afternoon, and we were like a bunch of giddy schoolboys impatiently trying to settle down and stand in line for the teacher after having just come in from schoolyard recess. Everyone had their packs with all their clean clothes, gear, and equipment. Many men carried cases of whiskey on their shoulders for the long road ahead—the road back to the war.

There were three planes taking us back to the war. Two of the planes were C-54s, a type of plane known as "the workhorse" during the Korean War. The C-54 is a four-engine, propeller-driven plane to which we were all very accustomed, always transporting the men and equipment back and forth, back and forth. We had all traveled this way a number of times and had grown quite weary of it. As I said, two of the three planes were C-54s, but the third plane was a new model, a C-117, referred to as "the flying boxcar." Every soldier desired to fly in the C-117. It was a two-engine box-shaped plane that you could drive a truck right into!

When the air policemen came, all of the soldiers tried to push their way to the front of the crowd right behind the rope so they could get a spot on the popular "flying boxcar." Luckily, I was in front of everybody else, so that I would be first to sprint out. The lieutenant ordered all of us to go to our own plane and then he dropped the ropes. Of course everyone rushed toward "the flying boxcar." Men were running and yelling to be the first in line to board that new plane. As we all ran, I was ahead of everybody else by a long way, especially because I wasn't carrying big cases of whiskey like many of the other men.

Inexplicably and all of a sudden, time slowed down all around me. It was like slow motion in a movie. My legs felt heavy. It was like a dream world, when you try to run but you can't, and no matter how hard you try, you keep feeling yourself falling farther and farther behind. I watched men pass me up, men who weren't even running very fast. "How strange," I thought. "What's wrong with my leg?" I wondered "What's going on?" Then I just slowed down completely. I thought, "Oh, well, I shouldn't be selfish." I knew everyone would get on one of the planes. The fuzzy, slow motion gradually started to fade and reality came back to me.

The air policemen yelled for us to get in a "column of ducks"—two columns. When men reached the plane, they started to form the lines, and I was toward the middle-back. Once we were all lined up, the lieutenant stood at the door and waved for the men to file in, counting as they boarded the plane. He allowed sixty of us on the "the flying boxcar," even though the limit was forty. Just as I was about to take a step onto the "the flying boxcar," this lieutenant slapped my chest and said, "All you from Jack on back have to take the C-54. This plane's full." We all groaned and complained angrily. I yelled, "Good grief!" still frustrated that I had inexplicably slowed down and ended up not making it in time.

Without delay, we hopped on the other airplane and flew to Korea. We landed in Chunchon, Korea. I thought it was odd because our original destination was Seoul City, Korea. Chunchon is about eighty miles inland from Seoul City. No one mentioned the reasons for landing in Chunchon though. Because we arrived in Chunchon, we then had to drive for a long time to get to our HQ (headquarters). We drove back in a two-and-a-half-ton truck and became dirty all over again. I unloaded and went to check in at the HQ tent at about 8:00 p.m.

It was a nice, clear summer evening; the sun was shining through the trees. When I got to the tent to check in, I saw my First Sergeant, Landon. He looked at me in astonishment and said, "Parks, you're here!" I replied, "Well, sure, I wasn't going to go AWOL." He repeated excitedly, "But you're here?" I didn't quite understand, so I just nodded my head and said, "Well, sure." "Did you hear about the flying boxcar?" Landon asked. "No," I replied. "What happened?"

He answered slowly, "It was circling to land at the Seoul City airport but crashed into the mountains next to it." He paused, then added solemnly, "There were no survivors."

"No kidding," I said quietly in amazement. "Do you know how close I was to getting on that flying boxcar? They allowed sixty men on that airplane, and I was number sixty-one!" I thought intensely for a moment. I was next in line to get on that plane, and I would have been killed. Then I remembered the experience I had trying to run to the airplane, how everything had slowed down. Suddenly, all the pieces came together for me, and I felt overwhelmed with gratitude.

"Well the good Lord was with me, because something kept me from getting on that plane," I told the sergeant gratefully.

Now I know that God had great plans for my life, and dying on the C-117 wasn't one of them. I am so thankful that I was protected that day; it was truly a miracle. I was able to go back home safely to my loving bride. God's grace is what I call it, God's grace.

•••

BIOGRAPHY: *Jack Parks, the third of six children, was born in 1929, in Stirling City, California. Parks determined early in his life to also become a pastor like his father. He attended Bethany Bible College but was drafted into military service during the Korean War. Honorably discharged in January 1952, he fulfilled his dream and became a pastor, while raising five children with "the love of his life," Ruby. Jack and Ruby recently celebrated their fifty-first wedding anniversary.*

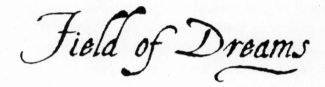

Field of Dreams

By Stephen Christopher Patterson

as told to his son, Kevin Patterson

At the age of only twenty-four—because I was told it would help my career path into flight school—I accepted a duty assignment in Okinawa, Japan, where I became the commanding officer of the Coast Guard LORAN Station, Gesashi. Gesashi is an island south of mainland Japan and is part of the navigational triad formed by the islands of Hokkaido, Iwo Jima, and Gelatin. These three communication stations by forming this triad provide navigational assistance in a 360-degree direction so that aircraft and ships have twenty-four-hour navigational assistance. During my two-week training prior to my taking command of the station, I was informed by the admiral of the Pacific fleet that I was going to be taking over a unit that had the worst performance record, had the highest drug and alcohol problems, and had the worst morale of any unit in the entire Coast Guard! Stunned by this revelation, I accepted the challenge because I thought I could, at the least, do as the admiral asked and "make some improvement."

The majority of the men stationed there had an age range from nineteen to twenty-four years old. My executive staff was men that were in their late thirties to early forties. So the challenge I had was that I was in charge of people who were roughly my own age and also people who were older than I. The biggest challenge was dealing with the executive staff that was not only older but also more experienced.

My style was that I liked to get as much input as possible from all people invited to contribute, take it under advisement, and then issue a decision. Once the leadership and chain of command were established, I was then able to start focusing on the operational aspects of the station. The main reason why performance had been poor was due to inadequate training and inadequate supervision, but most of all, it was due to inadequate pride. Pride is what makes individuals go the extra mile in order to do something that they wouldn't ordinarily do unless their boss was standing with them making them do it. By establishing pride in the unit, and a sense of accomplishment, the unit started to bond together, and it started to focus on a single purpose, which was to become the best unit in the entire Coast Guard in performance and efficiency.

Funny things happen once you get morale turned around and you get performance operating at a high level. It becomes a cherished item. My station became recognized for its great work, and everyone at the station took pride in that and they all felt like they had something to protect. For the last six months of my tour, I had 100 percent operating perfection, and that is something that had never been done in the entire history of the Coast Guard by any unit.

One of my main duties, aside from being a commanding officer, was to be in charge of the diplomatic relations between the Coast Guard and the local village on this island. It was necessary for me to introduce myself to the mayor of Gesashi and to his counsel so that they could be assured that the conduct and behavior of my men would continue to be of the utmost highest standards and that the people in their village would not have to worry about any misbehavior on the part of my men. It was also important for me to try to take the friendship and tradition that had existed in prior years between the mayor and the commanding officer to a higher level.

So when the mayor invited me to dinner and to watch sumo wrestling, I accepted. It is a privilege to be invited into someone's home. I was given the opportunity to learn their customs, traditions, and cuisine. I'd had such a good time that first time that the mayor invited me back the following week. My invitation into the mayor's home for dinner continued for weeks and weeks. Midway through my tour, the mayor informed me of the wonderful soccer team in the local village and also that the village had many boys who had a big interest in baseball. I told the mayor that I was a keen baseball player in high school and that maybe I could form a baseball team. I asked where their baseball field was—but the mayor informed me that the village did not possess a playing field.

The Navy Seabees construct airfields and do all types of bull-dozing, earthmoving, and large building construction. I had formed a very strong relationship with members of this unit. Since we were in war status, our particular unit had food and exchange privileges because we were more remotely located than the bases near Kadena AFB. The Seabees always had a shortage of grilled steaks and our unit had unlimited grilled steak privileges. So, on an island like this, there's a lot of wheeling and dealing—stuff like tires for steaks or file cabinets for gasoline.

I approached the commander of the Seabees unit and told him that we were trying to build a baseball field for the village of Gesashi. He agreed to bring a crew of men up and some heavy equipment and said it would take only one day! With their equipment and know-how, they were able to do huge amounts of work in a short amount of time.

They asked, "To what extent would you like this baseball diamond built?" We obviously needed a flat field that could drain, some back-stops and fences, dugouts and lights. They went to the Army disposition depot and collected up a lot of discarded cyclone fencing and piping, they found some lights, they brought up a load of concrete blocks. Early on a Saturday morning, they began. By Sunday night, they were totally done constructing this baseball diamond!

The diamond was dedicated to the village of Gesashi, and the mayor accepted it. After that, with a lot of sign language and arm waving, I was able to form a baseball team with the kids. It amounted to a team made up of ten- to twelve-year-olds. We got them ready for competition with other teams on the island.

Normally, when the military goes to foreign lands, the military will typically keep to itself. Obviously, it is usually there in an act of war or combat; there are often dangers associated with leaving base or your duty station. In this particular case, even though I was there supporting a war effort with the communications command, by the nature of the location on the island and the long, rich history of the relationship between the Coast Guard and Okinawa, we were able to more easily integrate with the people of the village. We helped enrich their lives, and they enriched ours.

They formed a baseball team and had a few games. They didn't do very well and I felt badly because they took the winning and losing very seriously. They felt that when they lost, they disgraced their village. Baseball, I explained, is played for fun; you win some, you lose some, and the rest get rained out. Toward the end of our season, they started to understand that there is always another game; if you lose a game, you just play another. So once the team got established, it was time to turn the team over to a local teacher who had played baseball.

As my tour came to an end in the summer of 1976, the mayor decided to hold a going-away party for my departure. It was held in the town hall and was attended by hundreds of people, including all the kids on the baseball team. I was presented a plaque by the mayor, with a letter written in their language on one side and another translated in English on the opposite side. As I stood there, I looked at all the people present and then saw the players. Within a few short days, I would be leaving the island—likely never to return. Even though a part of me was sad, a part of me was happy. I witnessed the positive results we'd achieved—a reward greater than any other.

My time was up in Gesashi, and my own dreams had been realized, too: I received word earlier that I had been accepted to naval flight school training in Pensacola, Florida!

A couple of days following the ceremony, I received notification that the admiral of the Pacific fleet was going to be making a visit to the station and was going to present an award. The admiral arrived and presented the station with a Unit Commendation medal. A Unit Commendation medal is for work above and beyond the call of duty. The admiral was greatly pleased not only by our performance and readiness, but also by the relationships established with the surrounding village and other branches of service with which we shared this island. Each and every person on that station received this award for excellent work. What makes this award impressive is that in a short twelve to thirteen months, this station went from being the absolute worst in the entire Coast Guard to the absolute best. Most of the men stood in total disbelief, but deep down inside, all of them knew how hard they had worked and the dedication it took to receive this recognition.

They say that war can make a man out of a boy, but I also think there are other experiences that can accomplish the same thing. Although I was twenty-four years old and considered a young man, I was probably still a boy at heart. And I will contend that those thirteen months during a war period made a man out of this boy. I learned a lot about what it takes to be a leader and the importance of being compassionate toward your fellow man. Also, I learned it is possible to change one corner of the world at a time without ever pointing a gun.

...

BIOGRAPHY: *Stephen Christopher Patterson was born in Seattle, Washington, in 1951. Upon his high school graduation, he received an appointment to the U.S. Coast Guard Academy in New London, Connecticut. After serving in the Coast Guard, he and his wife, Ginny, settled in California, where Patterson works in commercial real estate. He and Ginny have two teenage children: Kevin, sixteen, and Lauren, fourteen.*

Unlikely Evangelism

By Lyning Moore Peterson

In February 1969, the Vietnam War was in full swing and I was nine-teen years old. Ironically, those who did not want to end up there enlisted, providing themselves some small chance of staying out of 'Nam. Of course, if you wanted to further limit your chances, you def-initely avoided the Army, Marines, airplanes, and the medical field, so the previous December I'd enlisted voluntarily in the Navy's delayed entry program. On February 10, 1969, a mild, sunny winter morning, my parents drove me downtown to start my Navy enlistment, like mil-lions of other military personnel, at MEPS—the Military Entrance Processing Station—located in the U.S. Federal Office Building in the center of downtown Minneapolis.

Pulling his maroon Buick up to the curbside in front of the Federal Building, Dad stopped there for a quick drop-off and final good-bye, noting the parking was terrible and that he wanted to save himself the trouble. I think it was really for Mom's sake he did that, though, as her little one—I am the youngest of four—was leaving the nest and she did not like it. Having already said our good-byes at home, I shook Dad's hand from the backseat as he wished me good luck and leaned forward, meeting Mom for a quick hug. I stepped out of the car and, as I turned to walk toward the entrance, they pulled away.

I ascended the cold, stone steps outside between two groups of people. On the left, young men and women—"hippies" they'd have been called then—were handing out instructions on how to avoid the military and get to Canada. On the right, a group of men dressed in suits from The Gideons International, continuing their venerable tradition begun in World War II, were handing out pocket-sized, dark-green-bound copies of the New Testament with Psalms.

Armed with draft-dodging instructions in one hand and Scripture in the other, passing through this ideological gauntlet, I found garbage cans at the top of the stairs; those on the left were filled with draft-dodging instructions and those on the right with Bibles. Tossing the instructions away, I entered the building and found my way to the MEPS office. After waiting forever in a large room—they made us, a hundred-plus guys, strip naked to wait in one large room for our individual physical examinations—I took a physical that a dead man could have passed. Afterward, we were all sworn in to the U.S. armed forces and bussed to the airport to fly to our new home. The chartered plane hopped across the country toward San Diego, filling with new recruits at each stop. We finally arrived that evening, and two uniformed guys hustled us out of the plane, lining us up in two groups for our first of several roll calls.

After a short lecture regarding their expectations of us, the person in charge of the other group (it turned out he was a Marine) came over to our group and asked our leader (it turned out he was a Navy petty officer first class) how roll call went. He replied, "I got three extra."

The Marine said he was three short, to which the sailor generously offered in reply, "Take three of mine."

The Marine turned to our group and, facing in my direction, pointed to three recruits, one on my right, one on my left, and a third somewhere else. "You, you, and you," he barked, "get over there! You are Marines now!" The three left our group, and we never saw them again. Whether this was staged, I do not know; but it was the first of many lessons in scaring the "civilian"—plus some other stuff—right out of me!

After boot camp, the Navy immediately assigned me to a Seabee unit—a construction battalion, alias "CB" and hence the moniker. Since I'd graduated from a baking school, I skipped the Navy's "A" school where I would otherwise have gone to become a cook. I spent my first year with the Seabees, after which the Navy decommissioned the unit, and I went aboard ship, serving on the guided missile frigate, USS *Reeves* (DLG-24).

On the *Reeves*, I had primary responsibility for the storerooms and foodstuffs. Since I'd become a Christian after joining the Navy, during my free time I'd started a weekly evening Bible study, earning me the nickname "Preacher Peterson." With only three regular attendees, we really struggled to plant roots.

One morning in the middle of breakfast, just before leaving for a three-week cruise out of Pearl Harbor, my chief petty officer informed me I had forty-five minutes to bring aboard three weeks' worth of bread products, milk products, and fresh fruit or we'd sail leaving the load behind on the dock. The only way to get the stuff aboard in time was to pile it up on the mess deck, taking tables and seats away from sailors waiting to eat breakfast. Of course, everybody understood the necessary inconvenience and cooperated patiently; except for one, that is.

After we'd begun stacking all the produce, milk, and bread on mess deck, the mess deck master-at-arms, a higher-rated fellow cook—and a man prone to agitate when things did not go smoothly—came at me with a vengeance. Hyper-excited, arms flailing, he ordered me to clear my stuff out of the way. Keeping track of my time, my work detail, the food, and the master-at-arms was a trying task. Finally, he pushed one too many buttons, and I exploded. I remember feeling a part of me hanging back, objectively watching myself in shock while I tore into the master-at-arms with a fury of my own. The whole mess deck, everyone shocked, came to a standstill as "Preacher Peterson," a lowly E-4 (petty officer third class), verbally took apart that E-6 (petty officer first class) using language not fit for print.

When I'd finished, I turned and saw that right behind me stood my entire chain of command—the commanding officer, executive officer, supply officer, food service officer, and my cook chief—who had watched the entire encounter. Knowing my days as a member of the crew were numbered, I excused myself, went to the galley, and, entering the freezer, sat on a crate of frozen vegetables to contemplate life in a military prison.

Far from landing in the brig, however, it turned out that not only did my chain of command never say a word to me about the incident, but the master-at-arms was quietly removed and sent to another ship; unknown to me at the time, he'd had a history of similar behavior and this was apparently the last straw. That evening, the Bible study group exploded to thirty-five men and continued growing to a point where we had to divide into three groups.

And, by the way, all the food was aboard ship when we left port.

•••

BIOGRAPHY: *Lyning Moore Peterson was born in 1949 in St. Paul, Minnesota. After high school, he got a Baking Diploma at Dunwoody Institute and then enlisted as a cook in the U.S. Navy. After returning from Vietnam, Lyning earned his BA in accounting in 1978. Lyning and his wife, Joyce, whose two daughters are grown, now live in Harris, Minnesota. Currently employed as sign technician for the Chisago County Highway Department, Lyning also works part-time as custodian for his church and is a cook in the Minnesota Air National Guard with a rank of technical sergeant (E-6).*

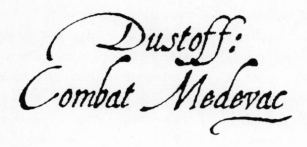

Dustoff: Combat Medevac

By Michael D. Rominger

At nineteen, I was sent to Vietnam as a warrant officer I (WOI) medevac helicopter pilot—a mission I chose, rather than just allowing myself simply to be drafted into who knows what, because I wanted my service to my country to mean something that reflected my values—because I wanted to save lives rather than take them. However, little did I know at the time that the mission of Dustoff—the Army's designation and call sign for medevac helicopters operating in combat—had a loss rate for pilots and crewmembers that made it one of the most dangerous types of aviation missions during the war. Slightly more than a third of the aviators became casualties in their work, and the crew chiefs and medics who accompanied them suffered similarly. Of all missions, hoists were the most terrifying and dangerous. One out of every ten enemy hits on the air ambulances occurred on such occasions, making hoists seven times as dangerous as the standard Dustoff mission. What follows is my account of one of my many hoist missions etched in my mind—a mission that may have been a little longer and more complex than most, but is otherwise not all that atypical for Dustoff. It shows what is routinely required of and displayed by every Dustoff crewmember every day, and it shows concretely the Dustoff credo of "When I Have Your Wounded." Dustoff crews (pilots, medics, and crew chiefs) were and are the bravest people I have ever known.

"Mr. Rominger! Mr. Rominger! Got a Mission! We've got a mission!" Fred, the Aussie medevac dispatcher, jars me out of a sound nap at 10:00 in the morning. I flew a three-hour patient transfer in the middle of the night and am a little tired. Mission sheet thrust outward in his hand, Fred bursts into our little wooden crew shack at Nui Dat—the Australian base in Phuoc Tuy Province just north of the port city of Vung Tau. I'm a "Dustoff" pilot—the term by which the Army designates its combat medical evacuation (medevac) helicopters—and here with my crew we wait for medevac missions.

John, my pilot, and Rich, the crew chief, are already sprinting to the aircraft. The medic, Mike, and I listen as the dispatcher gives us a quick rundown on the mission. "A LRRP"—Long Range Reconnaissance Patrol—"team of sixteen Aussies southwest of Xuan Loc has been ambushed. They're still in heavy contact with the enemy. They're surrounded, can't move, and already have six seriously wounded."

That area is all triple-canopy jungle, so I know it's going to be a hoist mission, as were most missions for the Australians and New Zealanders. "How in the hell did they let that happen?" I ask. Aussie LRRP tactics make it virtually impossible for a whole team to be ambushed; maybe a few team members, but not the whole team. With typical Aussie pragmatism he rejoins, "Don't know, mate, but I sure as hell know they need your help."

I grab the mission sheet and, heading for the aircraft, notice that it's short some information. "Who's my gunship support?" I yell over my shoulder. Company SOP (standard operating procedures) for good reason requires gunship coverage for all hoist missions; it would be virtual suicide without them. Hoists are our most hazardous mission, even with gunships, hovering for up to an hour in a hostile environment, unarmed—Dustoff teams comply with the Geneva Convention for medical operations and are therefore unarmed—at the tops of trees with a big red cross on the sides, the belly, and the nose of the aircraft.

"Can't find any yet, but I'll keep trying while you're en route!"

"Got it, see you on frequency." I throw on my chicken plate (armored chest plate) as John runs the throttle up to full RPM. Strapping in and putting on my helmet, I point to the west. Before I even have my gloves on, Mike and Rich each yell over the intercom, "In and clear," as John smoothly pulls on forty pounds of torque, swings the tail to the left, lowers the nose, and rapidly accelerates off the hospital pad. I can literally feel the power of the 1,400-horse-power turbine driving the transmission and rotors as it tries to torque the airframe.

As we accelerate upward into the bright, blue October sky—why do wars have to happen on such beautiful days?—I get on the radio. After checking artillery in the area to make sure we don't inadvertently cross someone's gun-target line at the wrong altitude, I check back with Fred to see who my gunship support is. "Everybody's tied up," he says. I start looking myself. The few "gun companies" whose frequencies I have can't help. So, going up on UHF Guard, the emergency frequency 243.00 megahertz, I make a request in the clear. "Dustoff three zero needs gunship support for a hoist mission at Yankee Sierra 235970." No response.

"Well," I think, "maybe the enemy has moved off and I can take a chance in hoisting out the wounded without gunships." Tuning up the LRRP team's frequency, I transmit, "Emu two six, Dustoff three zero, five mikes"—minutes—"out, what's your situation?"

In response, I get a very loud background noise—multiple machine guns, rifles, and explosions—and a stressed Aussie voice yelling, "Dustoff. Eight seriously wounded! Heavy contact, three six zero degrees! North flank in danger of being overrun! Can you take all sixteen of us?"

"Lord have mercy!" I think. No gunships, but I can't leave those guys there.

Another voice interrupts, "Dustoff, emu five six, come up 40.10." Dialing up 40.10 on the FM tactical radio, I call, "Emu five six, Dustoff three zero. Go ahead."

"We've been trying for air support all morning, but can't get any. How about you?"

"Sorry, no such luck."

"Figured as much. Those guys are in deep trouble. Any ideas?"

"Emu five six, who and where are you?" I ask.

"Dustoff three zero, Emu five six is Fire Support Base Coral. Do you have our coordinates?"

"Affirmative," I reply. "Five mikes out."

"Roger."

We land at FSB Coral. It looks like a scene out of Armageddon; trees, craters, piles of fertile earth, and howitzers are everywhere. The stares of hundreds of Aussie artillerymen greet me, the most concerned, pensive faces I have ever seen. As John runs through the shutdown and combat-cocking checklist, I walk toward the TOC (Tactical Operations Center).

An Aussie lieutenant colonel approaches me and, not wanting a sniper to recognize rank by a salute, I stick out my hand, "Hello." "This way, mate," he says, smiling, and leads me off to a briefing where we finalize a plan to save the LRRP team.

I am to orbit at two thousand feet a few miles east, while the team marks its position with smoke. Then, diving down to treetop level below the artillery, which will lay down a ring of fire around the team, a few seconds out of the hoisting area I will tell Emu to stop, hopefully timed so that I arrive just after the last shell falls. Bringing the aircraft to a hover over the team, I will tell them to resume their bombardment, hopefully keeping the enemy pinned down long enough to hoist out the team. While technically not gunship support, I hope the artillery meets the intent of the SOP, and more to the point, I hope it has the intended effect

Departing FSB Coral, I climb to two thousand feet and wait. Seeing green smoke filtering through the top of the triple-canopy jungle, I tell Emu and begin my dive to the extraction point. Flying into the wind, I slow to forty knots, put the collective pitch full down, and lower the nose to about –40E, placing the aircraft momentarily into a

½ G attitude and bringing our stomachs to our throats as the helicopter very quickly begins a three-thousand-feet-per-minute dive. As I G catches up to us, I begin a gentle left turn downwind toward the site. Just as I reach treetop level, about five seconds out, I key the mike and yell, "Stop!" Though the smoke has begun to thin, I have no trouble identifying the site—trees are falling and branches flying everywhere from the artillery barrage.

Yanking back on the cyclic and stomping on the left antitorque pedal, the aircraft very abruptly snaps 180E into the wind and I key the mike and yell, "Start!" Seconds later, the trees are disintegrating all around me again.

Gingerly, I begin nestling the aircraft into the treetops when the crew chief yells, "Penetrator on the ground!" referring to the hoist we'd just lowered. I was startled by the suddenness of his exclamation, because it was probably close to two hundred feet to the ground—but I wasn't going to argue with success. John closely monitors the controls with me—essentially both of us are now flying, an absolute requirement for combat because you never know when one of us is going to be out of the picture.

This is one of the most difficult types of flying I have ever done—with the aircraft nestled down into the treetops to get as much concealment as possible, I had to hold the aircraft perfectly still. This was a daunting task considering the wind and that the crew was moving around inside and sometimes outside onto the skids; the hoist out at the extreme of the aircraft's lateral center of gravity (CG); one, two, and sometimes three people on the jungle penetrator, hauling the people inside and moving them to different parts of the cabin—with the main rotor, tail rotor, and fuselage literally just inches from the tree branches, and sometimes while getting shot at. It required an extreme level of concentration and physical effort. Hoist missions always made you feel like you just ran a marathon while taking a college physics exam.

Five minutes pass, then ten, then—still hovering—all hell breaks loose. *CLINK! CLINK! CLUNK! BANG! TINK! BANG! CLUNK!* I can feel the rounds hitting the airframe. Some are unmistakably AK-47 rounds; others are heavier. I've been in more intense firefights, but not exactly like this; Rich and Mike are fully exposed on the skids while they hoist up the wounded and make sure we don't stick the main or tail rotors into the trees, and the helpless wounded hang suspended on the jungle penetrator. Dear God, why does that hoist take so long?

"One on board, gunshot to the upper right quad!" "Penetrator on the ground!" Five minutes. "Coming up, two on the penetrator, up, up!" "Three on board, head wound, looks bad!" Ten minutes. "Penetrator on the ground!" "Coming up, one on the penetrator, up, up!" Fifteen minutes. "Four on board, another head wound, looks bad, too!"

POP! POP! POP! (Rounds through the cockpit!) *BANG! BANG!* A round hits the back of my seat, right in the shoulder harness guide. It shatters and sends a bunch of fragments into my neck. There is blood everywhere. A second round misses my helmet by a fraction of an inch. The force of the round through the air slaps my head forward like I've been hit by a baseball bat.

John looks at me and sees the blood, and sees me slumped forward in my seat. We have a man just about to come up on the hoist, so he waits for a fraction of a second to see if he can bring him up. And then, suddenly, the instrument panel lights up like a Christmas tree! It looks like every red and yellow warning and caution light is lit up! That's all John needs to make his decision. He hits the "cable cut" toggle, pulls fifty-plus pounds (maximum) of torque, yells "STOP!" to Emu, and starts a hard turn toward Vung Tau.

John tells Rich I've been hit, and Rich pulls the seat-release levers on my seat, which tilts me and my seat backward. Rich and Mike pull me out of my seat, flop me onto my stomach, and start trying to figure out what has happened. Through my grimace I try to tell them what hurts, but Mike is already performing surgery on me.

John is talking to our unit and arranges for a replacement aircraft, but there are no replacement pilots. No problem. My injury does not appear serious, as long as no fragments have made it into the spinal column. We are now running on the battery, both generators are out, the hydraulics segment light is on, but the controls are merely stiff, so John thinks he can get it into the med pad.

Ten minutes later we land, leaking all over the place, at the 36th Evac hospital, and John does an emergency shutdown. The hospital staff pulls the wounded out of the aircraft, and our unit personnel meet us with a three-quarter-ton truck to haul us and our gear out to the new aircraft on the flight line. In less than five minutes, we are back in the air heading toward the LRRP team—with me wearing a large gauze pad on my neck.

Talking to Emu en route, I learn the situation is getting worse. This time I don't even bother with the standard "Dustoff approach" that I used the first time; three minutes out, I just put the pitch down and tell Emu I'm on approach. Again, as I reach treetop level, about five seconds out, I key the mike and yell, "Stop!" to Emu. Yanking back on the cyclic and stomping on the left antitorque pedal, I yell into the mike, "Start!" However, this time the *CLINK, CLANK, CLUNK* of enemy fire hitting my aircraft starts before I even get the aircraft settled into the treetops.

It's the same as before, directions from Mike and Rich to avoid hitting the trees, minutes passing likes hours, hoisting the wounded and taking enemy fire. I'm sweating and both arms are cramping now. Suddenly, *"BANG! BANG! POP! POP! POP!"* It's Christmas again! To my stupefaction, my right foot is suddenly under my seat, my left foot pushing hard on the left pedal, nearly slamming the tail rotor into the trees until John stops me from pushing it all the way forward. I can't see through the chin bubble anymore, except for a small hole in the center; something red is blocking my view—must be my blood. Boy, my foot hurts! John starts moving the aircraft out of the area, and I tell Emu "Stop! We're on our way out!" The artillery rounds stop right before we fly through their path. At least we got six more.

Rich and Mike want to pull me out of my seat, but I tell them no. It looks like I lost only the tip of my boot, so I tell them to keep working on the patients. Again arranging for another aircraft with a sarcastically miffed operations, we learn that there are still no replacement pilots. We land as before, and in ten minutes, we are back in the air—with me wearing a second large gauze pad, this one on my right big toe, which looks 25 percent smaller than before.

En route back I finally have time to ask how Rich is getting the penetrator on the ground so fast. I am answered by the slightly agitated voice of Mike, a more experienced Dustoff crew member than Rich, who says, "Sir, he reels out two hundred feet of cable inside the aircraft and then launches the penetrator out the door when you pull to a stop over the site!"

John and I just about have heart attacks! We explain to him the hazards of doing that—hitting people on the ground with the thirty-pound penetrator, kinking the cable so that it breaks, snagging equipment and/or people inside the aircraft and dragging them out the door, et cetera—and then thank him for his ingenuity but ask him to please not do it again. Whew!

Talking to Emu en route this time, they tell me the situation is critical—of the six people left, two are dead, which means there are only four combat effectives trying to hold off what is now believed to be at least a regiment of NVA (North Vietnamese Army regulars). Emu states that they have been virtually laying artillery on top of their position to try and hold the enemy at bay, but apparently, there are large numbers of them, and they are willing to risk extraordinary casualties to get at the remaining troops. I don't bother with the "Dustoff approach"—three minutes out I just put the pitch down and tell Emu I'm on my way in. The artillery barrage this time was significantly more intense and definitely closer. I yelled "STOP!" Just as I began to cross the line of artillery, I yanked back on the cyclic, stomped on the left antitorque pedal, and yelled into the mike, "START!" Immediately, *TINK, CLINK, CLANK* started. But Rich immediately yelled, "Penetrator on the ground!" God love that boy for disobeying orders! Five minutes. Ten Minutes. My legs begin to ache, but at least my right foot is numb.

"Two on board, KIA!"—killed in action. Good men, leave no one behind. "Penetrator on the ground!" Five minutes pass, then ten.

"Coming up, two on the penetrator, up, up!" "Four on board, last two only minor, arms and legs!"

"Penetrator on the ground!" Four minutes pass. God, I'm tired—arms and legs are both cramping. "Coming up, two on the penetrator, up, up! That must be the last of them, sir, because these two guys are shootin' the shit out of the woods below 'em!"

Over the intercom I ask, "Are there any branches in the way, or can I yank them straight up?"—a much faster way up than with the hoist only.

"Clear straight up! They're fifty feet below. Let's get the f—— out of here!"

BANG! POP! POP! POP! No lights this time; Christmas must be over. I pull on fifty pounds and hold the cyclic as still as I can. Rich yells, "They're clear of the trees," and I immediately lower the nose just enough to effect a rapid, level acceleration. I didn't want to start climbing to multiple thousands of feet yet, because I knew those guys hanging fifty feet below were probably terrified enough already, though probably happy to be out of the jungle.

"They're on board, no wounds!" Mike says. I look in back and see two slightly smiling, relieved faces. At that instant, all three of us glance at the two figures covered with ponchos lying on the litters. Smiling faces slowly turn grim, marked with tears. I turn around and begin a slow climb to two thousand feet.

I'm freezing to death because I'm soaking wet, and my arms and legs are cramped, so John takes the controls without having to ask. The med pad is a bit crowded, and we have only minor wounds, so we arrange for the KIA and us to be picked up at our revetment on the flight line, although this aircraft will need some maintenance, too, having taken nineteen bullets by my count.

Dustoff. Without using a bunch of clichés, I don't know how else to say it. Medevac pilots and crews love life and would do anything—ANYTHING—to save a life, including losing their own. With the bravery of these Aussies, or any and all of the troops I picked up during my year there, how could I do any less?

•••

BIOGRAPHY: *Michael Don Rominger was born in Ada, Oklahoma, on August 25, 1948. After serving in Vietnam, he pursued a career in law enforcement and fire fighting for the U.S. Forest Service, the California Department of Forestry, and the California Department of Justice, where he still serves today. A reservist, he was activated during Desert Storm, where he was the flight operations officer for the medevac detachment that supported General Schwartzkopf's "End Run" and led the medevac support for combat operations and postcombat operations in Kuwait. He and his wife, Roberta, have two grown children, Lynne and Matthew, and six grandchildren.*

The Water Rescue

By Colonel Dwight R. Rowland, USAF (ret.)

as told by his grandson, Brandon Rowland

I flew several types of bombers during World War II, the B-17, also known as the flying fortress, the B-24, and the B-25 Mitchell. The Japanese were holding an island some distance from the Philippines, where I was based. The island had a crescent-shaped harbor and our target was along the shore inside the curve. It was a short distance from the water to the target, and behind it were huge cliffs, which made it very difficult to bomb. We had to fly in and release the bombs even as we were starting to make a very steep turn to avoid the cliffs. As we were bombing, we were being attacked by antiaircraft fire.

On one mission, as we flew back to base, the stormy weather made it difficult to control my plane. I noticed then that one of our wings had been hit during the bombing run and fuel was leaking out of an engine. I knew I could get back on three engines, but shortly after I turned off the damaged engine, a fire began in an engine on the other wing. I cut off the fuel to that engine, and the fire went out. Now I was getting a little worried because going in on two engines would be difficult, and we might barely make it in.

About fifteen minutes later, a third engine went out, making the plane impossible to operate properly, and we had to ditch it. I yelled to my men to prepare to get out and radioed in our location. Losing altitude quickly, I looked at the water and saw waves at least three stories high. Ditching a plane in a storm is very hard to pull off; the plane must hit the surface in such a way that the waves do not overturn the aircraft. Although I had only one engine, I was still able to steer, if imperfectly. As we splashed into the water, I cracked my head on something and everything went black.

When I came to, the plane was still floating. I looked back and saw none of my crew. I assumed they had gotten out after we hit and must, therefore, be in our life raft. But then I noticed that they had not taken the life raft from the plane. I tried quickly to drag the raft through the plane to the escape hatch. I felt like I was in a boat, the plane rocking wildly back and forth. When I pulled open the plane door, a huge rush of salty water came flowing in, pummeling me and nearly tossing me into the ocean. The aircraft began to sink fast. As quickly as possible, I struggled to get the life raft out of the plane and onto the wing. Pulling the cord to inflate the raft and struggling to keep my balance as I got in, I realized the raft was attached to the plane with a rope. I tried to jerk it loose but could not. The sinking plane would soon pull the raft with it to the bottom of the ocean if I did not act quickly.

At a young age I learned always to carry a pocketknife for emergencies. So, hoping the force of the crash had not knocked it out, I reached into my pocket. Finding it, I pulled out the pocketknife and sawed through the rope, now underwater, cutting myself loose just as the plane disappeared under the surface and sunk rapidly to the bottom of the ocean. The wind, rain, and waves were almost unbearable, and the waves were a lot bigger even than I had expected. I looked around for all of my men and found that they were scattered at great distances one from the other in an almost semicircle pattern. My mind reeled. "Who should I rescue first?" I thought. I really wanted to get my best friend first, but as the captain, I could not play favorites. Deciding logically to rescue each person beginning with the nearest to me, I realized I did not have a paddle! If there had been one in the raft, it must have fallen out when it inflated. My only option was to paddle with my arms, one of the most tiring and difficult feats of my life. As soon as I paddled to the top of a swell, the wave would crash and send me back almost to where I had begun. When I finally did reach the first of my men and struggled to get him in the boat, I rejoiced inwardly in my success. Now, with four arms doing the work, paddling became easier.

When we reached the next man, one of my best friends, we found him hugging some floating debris. Severely wounded, his blood in the water around him. We carefully pulled him into the raft, but could not determine the nature of his injury since he could barely speak and the blood, awash over his entire body, obscured the wound. Though it took a very long time to accomplish, we continued to paddle from man to man, rescuing the entire crew.

For hours, we rode out the storm. When it finally subsided, we referred to an oceanic map one of the crew had grabbed from the plane, and found that the area in which we'd crashed was shark-infested. A little uneasy, we nevertheless calmed ourselves with the hope that if they did not get us while in the water, they would not get to us in the raft. For another day we floated with the currents until— quite literally out of the blue—the conning tower of an American submarine broke the surface of the water nearby.

Taking us aboard, they fed us and gave us medical attention—but too late for my wounded buddy. Because he'd gone well past the "golden hour" without medical attention, he died aboard the submarine. I later learned from the submarine captain that they had received the radio signal I sent during our crash. Heading toward the location where we went down, he spotted our raft through the periscope, which we had not noticed at all. Though grateful that most of us had survived the ordeal and were going to go back to our base, we nonetheless mourned the loss of a good man.

•••

BIOGRAPHY: *Dwight R. Rowland was born in 1917 in Robinson, Illinois. At college he met his wife, Barbara, with whom he had four children. Rowland joined the Army Air Corps in 1942 after graduating from the University of Illinois School of Law. After the war, he pursued a career as a judge advocate in the Air Force Judge Advocate General's (JAG) Department. Retiring at the rank of colonel in 1972, Rowland enjoyed "civilian life"—golfing, fishing, and visiting friends and family. He passed away in Sun City, Arizona, on April 15, 1991.*

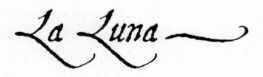

La Luna

Although I had served aboard the aircraft carrier USS *Hornet* during the Vietnam War, specifically in the Gulf of Tonkin, that was behind me for now and we'd made our way to the docks of Hawaii. The beauty of the Hawaiian Islands is something I find difficult to describe. It was especially beautiful after having just participated in maneuvers in Vietnam. The break to this exquisite locale seemed almost surreal to me. However, we were about to make history again.

The *Apollo 11* Lunar Landing Mission lifted off on July 16, 1969, from Kennedy Space Center at 9:37 a.m., carrying Neil Armstrong (commander), Michael Collins (command module pilot), and Edwin "Buzz" Aldrin (lunar module pilot). Everybody in America knew these names, riveted to black-and-white televisions as Neil Armstrong descended the lunar module ladder just prior to taking his first step on the moon. As he stepped onto the moon's surface, he proclaimed, "That's one small step for man, one giant leap for mankind."

Our role on the USS *Hornet* was to be there for splashdown in the Pacific Ocean 825 miles from Hawaii.

But stories were everywhere. It is kind of funny now. It was not funny then. It was, in fact, a little spooky. We'd heard that the astronauts might bring moon germs. No one had ever been to the moon and back before—and we didn't know what could happen. Moon disease was an unease that was very real to us. Nevertheless, we all got caught up in the excitement of the possible accomplishment for the United States—especially since there had been a lot of recent loss of life in Southeast Asia. The United States—the people of the United States and the soldiers all fighting—really needed the morale boost. The prospect of a successful moonwalk, germs or no germs, made everyone's spirits soar.

So, anyway, one of the greatest fears of the sailors was that the astronauts might infect us with some virus or disease from the moon. The dread we dared not think about though was the real possibility that these brave men might "burn up" upon entry. We just couldn't stand the thought that something might go wrong during reentry.

Then it happened. At 4:50 p.m., near Wake Island, the crew of the USS *Hornet* personally saw the capsule enter the atmosphere and descend toward the ocean. There was smoke. Then it hit the water as we held our breath; we could see on the horizon something was bobbing. Navy SEALs were sent out to pick up *Apollo 11* and the astronauts. We were only a few miles at most away from it all! It felt pretty exhilarating when that capsule hit the water and we knew Aldrin and crew were alive. The first men to have walked on the moon were coming on board our ship!

The Navy SEALs put a collar around the space capsule so it wouldn't sink. The astronauts were wearing biological isolation suits as a precaution against any "moon germs." First, the Navy SEALs pulled the astronauts out and they brought them into a decontamination center, which looked like a silver van in the middle of the carrier. The astronauts were quarantined because scientists—just like the sailors— didn't know if any diseases accompanied the spacemen. We could see the astronauts through the windows of the "van" and everyone was waving. Finally, we pulled the capsule up aboard and headed back to beautiful Hawaii.

Everything was offloaded from the ship. The capsule and the astronauts were all pulled off. Before we headed back out, President Nixon came aboard the carrier

Serving on the USS *Hornet* during the retrieval of the *Apollo 11* astronauts makes me one who has participated in one of the most incredible events of history. I just see it as serving my country. I don't feel I'm very important at all. After all, I didn't go to the moon—I just helped pick them up.

The hero astronauts enjoyed a ticker tape parade and a tour of twenty-five countries. We as a country were "over the moon" with excitement and success. Bittersweetly, however, our ship and crew that had retrieved the nation's heroes returned back to the Tonkin Bay and the war in Vietnam—a different duty, but no less important.

Appropriately, the USS *Hornet* is now a memorial to those who defended American values and to those who have pursued America's technological advancements. The aircraft carrier sits moored at Alameda Point in San Francisco Bay, close to where I now live. I'm proud to have been a part—albeit a small part—of the historic *Apollo 11* landing.

•••

BIOGRAPHY: *Victor Socrates Sakellar was born in Lynn, Massachusetts, in 1949. After graduating from high school, he enlisted in the U.S. Navy. Leaving the Navy in 1972, he began a career in the Merchant Marines. Living in the Philippines, he worked for the Defense Department, fueling cargo ships, while his help with Vietnamese refugees earned him an award from the Nixon Administration. Leaving the Merchant Marines in 1975, Sakellar started doing odd jobs and painting houses. He first started doing artwork in the early 1980s. Now making his home in Los Gatos, California, with his two dogs, Sakellar does odd jobs for local businesses and sells his paintings.*

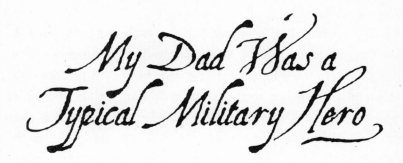

My Dad Was a Typical Military Hero

By Leo Scully

as told by Helen Scully

D ad was a military hero who buried his purple heart in his under-wear drawer. He rarely mentioned his service in World War II when I was a kid. While I did notice that Dad silently cried when he watched war movies and walked with a limp, I did not think much of it. It never really occurred to me to find out what he went through. It seemed to be an "off limits" subject. Now sixteen years have gone by since Dad died, and I wish I had asked him.

Last week I called my three older sisters and asked them what they could remember about Dad's military service. They could not tell me much. I also called one of my parents' best friends, Marie, who met my mother during the war in the unemployment line in Colorado Springs. She couldn't tell me much, either. "They didn't want to be singled out," she said. "If you made it through the war, you didn't want to talk about it." So, there are only fragments of information, pieced together fifty-eight years after.

My mother and father were married on January 31, 1942. A few months later, Dad went to Texas for basic training, and soon thereafter Mom joined him there and found out how big Texas roaches can really be. It was hot and far from home for two newlyweds from

San Francisco. Soon after, they went to Colorado Springs, where Dad completed Officer Candidate School.

I have no idea what happened between 1942 and 1944, but I do know that, in the summer of 1944, Dad landed in Normandy as an artillery lieutenant on Operation Overlord. He served in France for four months before his tour of duty was abruptly cut short. On September 4, 1944, Dad was in a jeep with four other men delivering payroll when they drove over a land mine. The explosion killed the others and threw Dad violently against a tree, shattering his hip and leaving him severely wounded.

Mom received the Western Union telegraph on September 21. Then twenty-five years old, Mom was alone in San Francisco raising my oldest sister, Lilly, who'd been born after Dad had already left. The message (which I still have, faded and yellow) says, "Regret to inform you your husband was seriously wounded in action four September in France." I can only imagine how Mom felt when she read those words. Like so many war brides, one of her worst nightmares had come true.

Traveling on the *Queen Mary* in a full body cast, Dad was transported to a hospital in California to be near Mom and my sister. Informed that he had a one-in-one-hundred chance of ever walking again, his recovery required extended immobilization—he was encased in plaster for a year and a day—followed by physical therapy.

The impact of Dad's injuries must have been staggering at first. Imagine, a newly married man in his mid-twenties raising a daughter while trying to grapple with the realities of a new, land-mine-affected life. Mom said he was never the same after the war. I think she felt she lost the man she married and was dealing with a stranger.

As it turned out, Dad did walk again, a testament to the depth of his courage and tenacity. Though he did walk, he suffered limited mobility; occasionally severe back pain debilitated him. He could not swing a golf club and generally sat on the sidelines of what would have otherwise been an active life. My sister Judy told me Dad had initially planned to be a contractor, using his hands and his strong body to make a living. But that dream was lost. Instead, he ended up at a desk job with the Internal Revenue Service as a middle manager until the day he retired. Dad had sacrificed greatly for his country.

Mom and Dad had good times and bad. Like many couples, they struggled to connect. Dad's experience during the war left a deep scar. Several years ago, before Mom died in 1997, she told me that she had a hard time communicating with Dad. She said it was lonely being married to a man you cannot reach. "He never got over it." she said. I think it is safe to say that Mom also paid a price for Dad's heroic contribution, and on some level the whole family paid a price. He was haunted.

But, while physical pain may have prevented an active life, it did not keep Dad from living a full life. He and Mom were a great team in many respects. Together, they raised four daughters and created a comfortable home on a middle-income salary. On weekends, they painted, refinished, and redecorated every room of our house. On Friday nights, they played a rousing game of bridge with friends. On Sunday afternoons, they yelled and screamed as Joe Montana charged down the field winning another game for the 49ers. The war was in the past and they didn't dwell on it.

When Dad finally got to retirement age, sixty, he was thrilled. That year, Mom and Dad moved from San Francisco and bought a house on the south peninsula where the sun shined and they had a view of the bay. As youngest and last child to leave the nest, when I turned eighteen and went off to college, I left them a brand-new empty nest and years to enjoy together. But, in that same year, open-heart surgery combined with the removal of his gall bladder put a major kink in Dad's retirement.

When he got out of the hospital, something had changed in Dad, for the better. He was more expressive. Maybe his heart surgery (and facing mortality) helped Dad recognize what was really important to him. His blue eyes twinkled with love as he enjoyed family time, interacting with his four daughters; his granddaughter, Julia; and his grandson, Charles. He lived eight more years after his quadruple bypass surgery. Then a violent case of viral pneumonia took him in less than ten days in 1986. He was sixty-nine years old.

Dad is remembered and admired by many, but especially by his grandson. Charles was inspired by my dad's military history and entered the Navy, following in his grandfather's footsteps. He is currently serving in the Navy and recently achieved officer status. As is appropriate, Charles has my dad's purple heart and the flag that was draped over my father's coffin.

In a few weeks, I'm going to Paris for the first time. We plan to visit the Normandy coast. I know I will feel my father's spirit there and will come to appreciate what he sacrificed in a much more personal way. He is not forgotten, and he is a reminder that my freedom has been earned. I try not to take it for granted.

•••

BIOGRAPHY: *Leo Scully served as a lieutenant in the Army in World War II in Europe where he was gravely wounded but survived. Scully worked for the Internal Revenue Service in various administrative capacities, including facilities management and security, for over thirty years. Husband to Marilynn and father to Lillian, Judy, Annie, and Helen, he is also fondly remembered by his granddaughter, Julia, and his grandson, Charles.*

Touched by History

By Rowleen Smith

as told to a friend

Vienna, Austria, in 1946 was not pretty, having been bombed heavily. Even though I'd seen pictures while stateside, when I arrived I could not believe how people were living. War's devastating effects were much more horrible in person. Their homes destroyed, the Viennese lived in structures without roofs as they dug out, day and night, remaking their world. Many wore burlap on their feet for shoes, and those who had something to eat at all ate black bread smeared with lard, sometimes only enough for lunch.

Not far from where I lived, there was a large, vacant lot. One day, strolling along the street in uniform, I found the lot encircled by a chain-link fence and behind it, hundreds of people. Most were elderly, although there were some children. A small sign on the fence read, in German, "Jewish refugees." These were Jews who'd been liberated from concentration camps and had no homes to which to return. This was to be a temporary place for them to await transportation to somewhere for permanent settlement, to begin rebuilding their lives. Their clothes were in shreds, and they looked pretty bad. Despite their numbers, they were very quiet. As I stood there gawking at them, a few noticed me and approached the fence. An elderly man beckoned to me to come over to him, and I did. He asked me in German, "Are you Jewish?"

"Yes," I said.

He poked his old fingers through the chain-link fence so he could touch my uniform. He was crying and looking at me, and as he kept rasping softly with emotion over and over again, "Amerikanische, Amerikanische, Amerikanische!" I stood there, weeping. The rest started crowding toward me and poking their fingers through the fence to touch me. They were crying. I was crying. Only two days later, they were gone, having left for a permanent settlement location.

Meanwhile, in contrast to the devastation and homelessness, the building in which I was billeted was a beautiful, unique two-story building across the street from a shrine to Mozart. German SS troops lived there before the Soviets captured Vienna in April 1945. Some of them had carved their initials and what I assumed were names of hometowns on the wooden window frames. The building's entry-level floor was of glass brick, through which people in the basement dining facilities could look up from their meals and see the feet of people walking on the floor above. Notwithstanding the building's architectural anomaly, I usually breakfasted in the mess at the top of the Austrian Bank Building where I worked, another gorgeous building, where they offered a larger menu.

I could order anything I wanted there, from steak and eggs to simply coffee and toast. Interestingly, no matter what you ordered there, even if only coffee and toast, the Viennese staff would bring steak and eggs, sausage, hot cakes with syrup, fresh fruit, and, of course, the coffee and toast. If you said, "I didn't order that," they would apologize, "I beg your pardon, madam" or "I beg your pardon, sir," then throw your silverware in the middle of the tray of food. Then all that unordered food would get dumped into a five-gallon drum and at night they would take it home for themselves. Everybody knew; nobody said anything.

One time I was on furlough somewhere—my memory fails me on the specifics—during my tour in Vienna, traveling by military train.

Though at the time there were no dining cars on the trains, each train stop had a mess hall so soldiers traveling away from their billets would have a place to eat. At one of these stops, I got off the train to eat. In the middle of my table was a huge bowl of fruit. Even I, a Californian, was impressed at the mammoth size of two particular oranges in the bowl. After my meal, as I left I scooped them up for a snack on the remainder of my trip.

Exiting the mess hall, I waited for the next train, holding an orange in each hand, standing several feet from a local woman and her son, who appeared to be about five years old. Though distracted at first, when I noticed them, the mother was tugging lightly at the little boy, who, transfixed, stared, pointing toward me. He wasn't staring or pointing at me, though. His huge eyes, incredulous, were locked on the two oranges. The poor, thin mother looked a little embarrassed as she tried to calm down her son. No longer distracted, I found myself riveted by him.

After a few moments, I approached them, the mother looking anxious. Smiling, I slowly held out the two oranges to the little boy and he gasped. His warm, tiny fingers touched mine as he reached out to accept the oranges and, taking them, began to cry as he held the fruit to his nose and smelled them. Before I could stop her, the mother dropped to her knees and actually kissed my shoes over and over again. As she rose, she rubbed her face on the back of my hands, sobbing.

Almost four decades later, I can still feel the electricity of that incident. Every moment of that brief exchange is etched in my mind, and the sound of the little boy's big gasp is as clear and audible today as it was then.

I shall never forget the sights, sounds, smells, and feel of the little boy's warm fingers and the gnarled, aged hands of the old man reaching through the fence, the mother kissing my shoes with tear-stained lips, and the sea of faces behind the chain-link fence, weeping with me as they reached out to stroke an American military uniform. In these incidents, which continue to reach out to me across time, I was touched, literally, by history.

•••

BIOGRAPHY: *Rowleen Smith was born Rowleen Goldberg in Philadelphia, Pennsylvania, and grew up in southern California. After graduating from high school, Smith enrolled in Los Angeles City College to study drama but left to join the Army in 1944. Trained as a medic in the Army, Rowleen served at Letterman Hospital in San Francisco until 1946, when she reenlisted for an assignment in Vienna, Austria, where she served until 1948. A retired cytologist and mother of two adult sons, she currently resides in Ventura, California.*

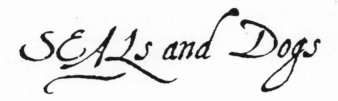

SEALs and Dogs

By Mike S.

as told to Scotty Daniels

On one of my twelve missions in Afghanistan, my team unloaded on al Qaeda members at Tora Bora. We infiltrated fifteen cave complexes and the largest al Qaeda training facility in Afghanistan. Using a million pounds of explosives and bombs, we obliterated the entire area. My platoon used more bombs in our first week in Tora Bora than were used during the first six months of the Vietnam War. We killed hundreds of Taliban and al Qaeda troops. There was only one living creature left, a puppy. Although hundreds of enemy troops had perished, the lonesome mutt was still standing.

Hot and smoky, the desert reeked of death. We could not help smiling at each other when we saw the pup, though. He looked about three months old, a little like a German Shepard but with long, droopy ears. He was very skinny and obviously hungry and thirsty. Cautiously, we approached him. He was scared to death, shaking with fright. When he decided we were friendly, his little tail started to wag. All of us were gathered around him, petting him. Now really excited, he started to run in circles.

From that moment, it was like having a little bit of home nearby. I felt good. The pup followed our ten-man platoon back to camp.

Arriving back at camp, we gave him one of our MREs (Meals, Ready to Eat), which are usually very disgusting, but not to this little thing. He gobbled it right up. It was probably the best meal he's ever had. Of course, we had to name him. Our lieutenant, Lieutenant C., decided to call the pup JDAM—pronounced "Jay Dam," shorthand for Joint Direct Attack Munition, a guidance system used to convert general purpose free-fall bombs into guided "smart" bombs—and our entire platoon took to calling this homeless mutt by that name. Sheltered and loved, he became part of our platoon. Whatever missions we went on, he was there. Whatever we ate, he ate. Whenever we slept, he slept. This mutt was like an alert system ready to help out his newfound friends.

A few months later, the U.S. Navy veterinarian was making his rounds caring for the U.S. K-9 units in Afghanistan. We told him about JDAM and asked whether he could give him the vaccinations required by the Navy so we could bring JDAM home with us to America. He agreed and gave the pup his shots, the newest and smallest member of the Navy SEALs.

In May, we finally got orders to return to the States. JDAM boarded the plane with us as one of the guys. He had been through it all. Although our commanding officers did not find out about JDAM while we were in Afghanistan, they later saw pictures and read articles in newspapers about him.

JDAM now lives with my friend, Lieutenant C., and his family, and every once in a while, I pile my kids in the car and we all go to visit him.

●●●

BIOGRAPHY: *Mike S. was born in 1967. In 1990, just five years after graduating high school, he enlisted in the U.S. Navy and became a Navy SEAL. The next twelve years were spent serving his country in many highly confidential missions. He left the Navy in 2000 as a petty officer first class to pursue a career in fire fighting, but also signed up for the Naval Reserves. In December of 2001, he received orders to return to his Navy SEAL platoon and was immediately sent to Afghanistan. Raised in southern California, Mike is happily married to his wife, Susie, of thirteen years and has four children ranging from two to twelve years old.*

A Leader of Marines

—— By Captain Andrew Unsworth, USMC (ret.) ——

as told to Milo James

On August 15, 1968, I transferred to my first grunt unit since arriving in-country in May, 3rd Battalion/26th Marines (the "3/26"), at Phu Loc 6, just south of Phu Bai on South Vietnam's northern coast. The 3/26 was then providing road security over a twenty-mile stretch of Highway One. In the late afternoon of my first day in the bush with Lima Company, my platoon, enjoying some downtime, was sitting around on the crest of a hill.

One guy near me busied himself absentmindedly, spiraling upward and then catching with a casual familiarity an M-406 grenade, much as one might do with a football. The spherical M-406, fired from the M-79 grenade launcher, would not detonate merely on impact. Instead, designed to arm itself about fifteen meters downrange after being launched at seventy-five meters per second doing thirty-seven hundred revolutions a minute, the grenade arms itself after about twelve revolutions. Only then would it detonate on impact.

Having noticed this, I made a show of standing up and theatrically taking five giant steps away. Somebody asked what the hell I was doing. "Well," I replied, nodding toward the grenade, "if that thing goes off cuz it's spun enough times to be armed, I don't wanna be in the kill zone." That hit home, and much more diplomatically than had I, the new kid, tried to upbraid the guy for complacency.

Thus orienting myself to my first grunt unit, I fit in pretty well. A few months later, we joined a half-dozen other Marine battalions a week before Thanksgiving for Operation Meade River, which 1st Marines had planned and directed in connection with the Le Loi pacification campaign. Its goal—as this lowly PFC understood it—was to weed out Communists from among the local population and destroy the local Vietcong infrastructure. Beginning the morning of 20 November, the seven Marine battalions cordoned off a thirty-six square kilometer area of lowland rice paddies and fields, in an area we called Dodge City, and gradually contracted the cordon until victorious.

All night, a number of AC-47 and/or AC-119 gunships—I could not see them so I don't know which—flew overhead parachuting flares over the cordoned-off area, timed so that when one burned out another replaced it. I could make out the box pattern in which the planes flew by the orange-red incandescence of I-don't-know-how-many floating flares. Though bright enough to have read by, the flares, floating under parachutes, cast eerie shadows on the ground that shifted randomly, playing games with my mind.

One night, when my platoon had point, I was sloshing through the rice paddies—one can't easily tiptoe quietly here—humping a PRC-25 radio on my back and carrying my M-16 rifle, the smell of human and animal fertilizer ripe in my nostrils. Suddenly, we started taking light machine-gun fire from a bunker and I dropped. Belly down, my head and radio above water, I looked up. Green phosphorescent tracer rounds zipped overhead all around us. For a moment I thought (strange as it sounds) how beautiful they looked. Slightly behind me to my left, a Marine with an M-72 LAW (a lightweight, disposable antitank weapon) telescoped the tube-shaped weapon open and armed it. I watched his silhouette as he stood, facing the offending fusillade, and placed the weapon on his shoulder. To my horror, and then astonishment, an instant before he fired, a tracer round pierced the front of his helmet and exited out the back. Staggering slightly, he squeezed the trigger bar. The LAW's conical backblast whooshed outward as the rocket shot downrange, and he splashed back into the rice paddy, unharmed. Apparently, he'd tilted his helmet back in order to take better aim, and in so doing, pushed it upward far enough that the bullet merely gave him a haircut.

Other Marines did not fare so well. Though the operation accomplished its objective, it came at a cost—over one hundred Marines gave their lives and several hundred were wounded. In return, however, the Communists lost over eight hundred, and Marines took almost two hundred prisoners, not including the capture of most of the Vietnamese who'd formed the Vietcong infrastructure.

Not long after Meade River, the 3/26 stood down for reconfiguration. Since I did not have much time left in-country, I transferred to 3rd Battalion, 5th Marines (the "3/5"). Having developed a not-atypical tribal worldview of the Marines, I found myself a bit critical of the way the 3/5 operated versus the way we'd done things in the 3/26. However, a buddy who transferred with me admonished me to be patient. So inclined, on about my third day with the 3/5, we began running patrols in forestlike terrain of the Que Son mountains. While on a platoon-size patrol, another squad had point. That squad's point man—a confident, wiry little guy, built like a greyhound—made his way through the bush, his gloved hand wielding a machete. We'd been out all day without having made enemy contact when, as it began to rain, I realized we hadn't rotated the point squad, nor had the point squad rotated its point man. (Rotating the point man is good for a few reasons, including spreading the risk inherent in taking the point and ensuring the point man is fresh, both mentally and physically.) We were close to heading back, when a resonating *BOOM* sounded from in front. The point man had tripped a booby trap.

Fortunately, though wounded, he didn't die. The rest of the column spread back down a side trail on the sloping hill while our corpsmen tended to his injuries. We carried him out from there, several of our bigger guys taking turns. Moving along the trail, I noticed along the side three fairly inconspicuous formations of three rocks or sticks each, alternately parallel and perpendicular to the trail. Stopping the Marine behind me, I pointed them out.

"Yeah, so?" he said.

I'd learned back in Camp Pendleton that the enemy used such formations as indicators of nearby booby traps; apparently the word hadn't spread to all units in-country.

This booby trap incident served as a sort of epiphany for me, a watershed moment that, in effect, determined the rest of my life. Realizing there was just too much for any one person to learn, I decided then I'd like to stick around, to make the Corps my life and impart what little knowledge I have to others. So, after Vietnam and duty in Okinawa, I went home to Indianapolis, where, while attending Indiana University, I completed the Marine PLC (Platoon Leader Course) program. After graduating, I was commissioned a second lieutenant in the U.S. Marine Corps, where I am proud to have spent the next twenty-one years as a teacher and leader of Marines.

•••

BIOGRAPHY: *Andrew Unsworth was born in 1949 in Indianapolis, Indiana. In September 1967, Unsworth enlisted in the U.S. Marine Corps. During his Marine Corps career, Unsworth achieved the ranks of both first sergeant and captain. He later attended Indiana University and currently serves as a project manager for a general contractor. Unsworth and his wife, Nanellen, have two daughters and a son.*

A Ministry of Presence

By Chaplain (LCDR) Diane Wilson, USN

as told to Milo James

U.S. Naval Station Guantánamo Bay, 1992. I could not believe I was actually there. Looking at the sea of Haitian faces under the hot Cuban sun on either side of the pickup truck as we drew nearer to Camp Buckley, I thought, "What can I possibly give these people in this desperate state of affairs?" Not merely boat people, these 233 would-be refugees (out of thousands of Haitians in other nearby camps) at GTMO—shorthand for Guantánamo and pronounced "gitmo"—were also HIV positive. "I could be watching this on CNN at home," I thought. "Yet, here I am." I realized, now in a very surreal but undeniable way, God had opened to me the opportunity to serve a special third-world ministry through a mechanism I'd never in a thousand years have predicted.

Pondering the events that resulted in my participation in Operation Able Manner/Safe Harbor, I could only ascribe it all to my Lord. While my path to military service from social work had been dubious enough, as a very green Navy chaplain, I found myself assigned, of all places, to a Marine unit. A former assistant pastor from Stockton, California, and social welfare worker from San Francisco's Fillmore district, I was at first certain the Marines were going to have me for breakfast. However, I survived long enough to make this first of two overseas deployments with 2nd Medical Battalion, 2nd Force Service Support Group, six months after arriving at Camp Lejeune. And long enough to learn that, despite their well-deserved reputation for ferocity on the battlefield, the Marines were also overwhelmingly devoted to God and country with a lamentably underreported compassion.

As I passed through the Haitian multitude, I presented to their curious eyes an apparent paradox: the pectoral cross of a Navy chaplain worn outside a camouflage military uniform. The desperate Haitians did not understand these things at first, of course. The uniform, after all, represented the military power that, having first rescued them from the treacherous Caribbean, now detained them, foiling their attempt to reach America with its promise of a better future. Yet, by that cross they thought they found in me a savior from this frustrating—if beneficent—crucible. Having fled Haiti in the wake of the September 1991 overthrow of Jean-Bertrand Aristide, these refugees were among tens of thousands seeking fulfillment of a desperate hope. Risking their lives, they traveled in small, crowded boats and rafts, weathering storms that drowned many; they watched (or heard the terrified shrieks of) family and friends devoured by sharks; and they suffered under the scorching sun, until rescued by the U.S. Coast Guard, all in the attempt to make a home in the United States.

Soon after I arrived, my command chaplain, recognizing, of course, that Camp Buckley was a special camp, gave me a day to consider taking the assignment. But to me, working there was a fait accompli; it was very clear to me that God had worked together all things to bring me here. I gave my "RPI"—Religious Programs Specialist First Class, a noncommissioned officer—the same chance to consider accepting this opportunity as my command chaplain had given me. But, like me, he was readily receptive, and together we committed ourselves to going forward, unequivocally, as a team.

My second hurdle was more difficult; in fact, it was in part outside my control. Though not one to apologize for my gender, neither am I much of a feminist. I was, therefore, both keenly aware of the patriarchal Haitian culture and free of any ideological ego prompting me to be "in charge." So prepared, I began my ministry with the initial goal of merely being seen; of allowing the people, and especially the Haitian pastors—also HIV positive—to get a sense of who I was, of engendering in them comfort that I was not there to interrupt or pursue a personal agenda. Knowing my first open door would be the Cross, I made it my business to seek them out and establish a rapport, a bond of mutual respect.

I did not know whether the Haitian pastors were credentialed or simply moved by the Spirit to fulfill a powerful need, nor did I care. For when all else fails for a people in such a state of disarray, helplessness, and despair, their mainstays are their hope and faith in God. Knowing, then, that relating to them would be through that medium, in aligning myself with the camp pastors, I made sure my only motive was to be open to their needs. Working through interpreters and learning simple Haitian Creole phrases and the power and finesse of body language, I connected, assuring them my presence meant support, not spiritual (or other) hegemony.

Officially, of course, my role was to liaise between the military command structure and the camp, providing a sense of the camp climate and communicating official information to the Haitians, and to assist in distributing food, clothing, shoes, toiletries, books, and other necessities. More important, though, was my "ministry of presence"—just being there. I spent many sixteen- and eighteen-hour days not only in worship services, distributing goods, and serving meals, but also "ground pounding," walking a beat over the sun-baked ground through the ad hoc village of temporary shelters—the Navy Seabees erected pressed-wood shelters on cement foundations, which, while not fancy, were nonetheless sturdy and relatively comfortable—making myself available. Sitting with the refugees on their cots, through interpreters I offered what I could. Whether counseling or listening to the dreadful stories they needed to tell, or holding their hands and merely sitting quietly listening for that "still, small Voice within," I did my best (I hope) only to be present, in the present.

After a time, I noticed the phases the Haitians went through. Initially struggling with the tension between the Cross, on the one hand, and the uniform, on the other, they then alternated their focus from what they perceived to be my role as savior to my role as representative of the U.S. military. Ultimately, though, the bonds of trust and love that developed pared away the inaccurate and superfluous, and this ministry of presence began to produce a quiet fruit. I began to see in these men, women, and children much more than their wretched social and political status and frightening medical condition; I began to understand the real and meaningful benefit of their faith, especially during worship.

In their worship services, they drew heavily on the Psalms, which, I think, spoke their language. Pregnant with lamentation, hope, and faith in ultimate spiritual victory, the Psalms speak to a people oppressed, crying out to and hoping in a Lord, who—in the final analysis—will not forsake them. Like the comfort the Psalms provided, music also was a refuge for them. In particular, and with special poignancy, they found solace in Scriven's well-known hymn, "What a Friend We Have in Jesus." Hearing them sing the familiar song (written by a nineteenth-century Irishman) in their own language, I thought them absolutely angelic. Moved deeply, I viewed the scene as a wondrously touching expression of the substance of their hope, the "evidence of things unseen."

My participation in this deployment taught me the fullness of what the chaplaincy offers, showed me that—so far from a marketing slogan—what I did and do in the Navy really is an adventure, not just a job. An opportunity unlike that available though any other vehicle, the Navy chaplaincy has provided me the chance to minister to the destitute, the homeless, the sick and dying, while simultaneously serving God, country, and fellow servicepersons. The military has sent me to places I never thought I'd see and, in particular, afforded me the opportunity by this third-world ministry the chance to see the Psalms come alive.

...

BIOGRAPHY: *Born in 1954, Diane (Cromer) Wilson received her under-graduate degree in Social Welfare from San Francisco State University in 1977 and her Master of Divinity degree in 1983 from San Francisco Theological Seminary. Commissioned in the U.S. Navy in 1991 and married in 1994 to Blane Wilson (currently a Navy captain), Wilson now serves as the Protestant chaplain to the servicemen and servicewomen at NTTC Corry Station in Pensacola, Florida.*

The Orphanage

By John Witwer, M.D.
as told to Chelsea Short

Vietnam, 1967. I arrived in-country in October, more than two years after the United States sent its first combat troops to Vietnam. I was a doctor and a captain in the U.S. Army, full of conviction about joining the fight against the spread of Communism. Recently graduated from Cornell Medical School and having completed my internship, I'd volunteered for military service because I sincerely felt that Communism was ultimately destructive to the United States and I did not want to see my country harmed by its further expansion. After my arrival in Saigon, my unit, the 210th Combat Aviation Battalion, was sent to an area near the small town of Long Thanh, where we established our camp. Also near Long Thanh, in a Special Forces camp, Green Berets and other agents trained for running operations into North Vietnam, Laos, and Cambodia. As battalion surgeon, I treated our soldiers and civilians, though, despite my title, I really didn't perform many surgeries; I was simply a doctor who took care of the troops.

The Dao-Dong Buddhist monastery had established an orphanage in Long Thanh approximately two miles from our camp. The orphanage was a branch of the monastery, and the bonzes and bonzesses—

Buddhist monks and nuns—cared for children who had lost their parents in the war. Many of them were orphaned because the Communists had murdered their mothers and fathers, in particular those who were doctors, lawyers, teachers, journalists, and other members of the "intelligentsia."

In addition to our regular duties, my unit and other local units went out to help at the orphanage once or twice a week, where there was plenty of work for us to do. As an M.D., I would do a "sick call" for the kids. Dressed in long, saffron robes, heads shaved, they would come to me with runny noses or infections, scrapes or bruises, and I'd treat them. I even wrote a handbook for the orphanage concerning the treatment of their ailments and the usage of medications. Meanwhile, my then-girlfriend, Jean (whom I later married), would send us much-needed supplies for the orphans from home. On the monastery's land, there was a small farm, and the children were taught how to cultivate the soil for growing their own food, for it was important that the kids learn how to be self-sufficient. The children liked to play organized games, and so we played with them. I recall in particular the children playing one Vietnamese game, reminiscent of what we know as ring-around-the-rosy, and to this day I can see their smiles and flowing robes and hear their laughter. No matter what they were playing, though, the most important thing to the children was that they were playing together. Though attired completely differently from Western children, a six-year-old's smiling face with two missing front teeth is the same in any culture, and in that context was symbolic of the reason I served in Vietnam.

In spite of the bonds formed, however, we could not truly converse with the kids because none of them could speak English, and Vietnamese was an incredibly difficult language for us to learn. The slightest change in tone of voice, the most minuscule variant of pronunciation, could mean the difference between two completely different—though to us, identical sounding—words. Whenever I attempted to speak to the kids in their native tongue, they would look at me with blank stares, and I knew I had said something wrong. With the adults, however, we spoke in a patois of Vietnamese, English, and French. Communication in this ersatz language was difficult, but we made it work.

The man in charge of the War-Born Orphan Village, as it was called, was named Nguyen Van Su. A Buddhist priest who radiated an almost palpable inner peace, Mr. Su was one of the most quietly charismatic people with whom I have ever come into contact. He spoke fluent English, and I became very close to him in the time that I spent at the orphan village. Mr. Su refused to accept money or handouts, but was nonetheless deeply appreciative of our help with the children. I remember distinctly Mr. Su telling me, "John, tell us how to do things, because someday you'll be gone." We followed this request and taught Mr. Su and the monastery's bonzes and bonzesses what we knew, helping them to help themselves.

In Vietnam at that time, one could not tell for sure who was an enemy and who was a friend; some of the Vietnamese helped the Americans by day and the Vietcong by night. Therefore, we could never really know for certain which side Mr. Su was on, but he loved the children so much and we'd come to trust him so completely that the subject of his political sympathies was trivial. It did not matter to us at all.

When I returned home from Vietnam, I tried to contact the War-Born Orphan Village but stopped after six months of no replies. A friend of mine who went to Vietnam several years ago tried to locate the orphanage, but he didn't have any success, either. My guess would be the antireligious North Vietnamese regime shut down the monastery some time after they took over Vietnam. While I would not be surprised if my friend Mr. Su had ended up in a "reeducation" camp, in the end, sadly, I really have no way of knowing what became of Mr. Su or the orphanage.

Before I left Vietnam in 1968, the orphanage honored some of its benefactors. I was one of many to whom, in a sublimely poignant ceremony, they paid tribute. The bonzes and bonzesses gave me flowers and a medal and the children sang and danced. Although the Army did not give me any official award or recognition for my work at the War-Born Orphan Village, the admiration from the adults and children there was the most touching prize I could have possibly received. I truly miss them.

...

BIOGRAPHY: *John Witwer, M.D., was born in 1949 in Pittsburgh, Pennsylvania. After studying pre-med at Amherst College, Witwer graduated from Cornell Medical School in 1966 and volunteered for Vietnam. After returning from Vietnam, Witwer had a private practice in Wheat Ridge, Colorado. He retired in 1996 and began a career in politics. He currently serves the people of District 25 in the Colorado State House of Representatives. Witwer and his wife have two grown children and reside in Evergreen, Colorado.*

On the Tip of the Spear

— By Captain Paul Michael Wojcik, USMC (ret.) —

When Iraq invaded Kuwait, I was the electronic warfare officer in the operations office of II MEF (Second Marine Expeditionary Force) in Camp Lejeune, North Carolina. Since the Marine Corps had tasked I MEF for the Gulf War and many units needed forward air controllers (FACs), I volunteered for FAC duty with I MEF. After FAC School, I shipped out to Saudi Arabia, arriving in-country on January 30, 1991. After I went through in-processing at the Port of Jubail, I was assigned to the 1st Marine Division at Manifa Bay, where, after a few days, they decided to send me to the 1st Light Armored Infantry (LAI) Battalion—appropriate in a poetic way since 1st LAI's motto, "Tip of the Spear," described my job as a FAC pretty well.

My first morning at LAI headquarters was clear and cool. Assigned to Charlie Company about three klicks (three kilometers) from the Saudi-Kuwaiti border, I hitched a ride from HQ to my new company. After being introduced to my company's Commanding Officer (CO) and exchanging pleasantries, I boarded an LAV-C2 (Light Armored Vehicle, Command and Control)—a turretless, field-command station resembling a desert-camo-painted shoebox on eight knobby tires—and went to OP-5 (Observation Post 5) on the northern Saudi-Kuwaiti border to call in my first mission, an aerial attack from two AV-8B Harriers.

Visibility was good; I could see my target, a police station used as an Iraqi forward observer position, about a kilometer across the border. Standing on a seat inside my LAV, exposed from the waist up, I radioed the lead Harrier. After giving him his brief and laser codes, turning on the laser and getting his confirmation, I gave him his vector to target, and "cleared him hot." His two-thousand-pound laser-guided bomb tracked on target then broke lock and went stupid, blowing up near the police station without hitting it. The next Harrier experienced a similar problem, though the sorties had the desired effect, as we took no more artillery or rocket fire.

That was the first time I ever tried to take a human life. I knew I had to just do what needed doing, but although from the waist up I operated smoothly, crisply, even academically—the result of good training—below, my knees shook uncontrollably. After that orientation to combat, doing what had to be done, though often frightening, was mainly business as usual.

Several days later, we repositioned to OP-3, where, earlier, Delta Company, First LAI, had battled two Soviet-built T-54 tanks that were part of an Iraqi flanking maneuver during the Battle of Kafji. Interested in the effectiveness of a TOW (Tube-launched, Optically tracked, Wire-guided) missile on a T-54, I climbed onto one of the tanks. The tank's turret had been blown off, landing askew of its carriage, exposing the interior. Inside, it looked like a blender had minced the tank's innards—burnt shell casings, shards of metal and bone lay all over the place. On the scorched driver's seat sat a pile of vertebrae; the rest of the driver was gone. Outside, the remains of the tank's commander (he'd been thrown from his hatch) lay in the sand. I'd never seen anyone burned before, and hope never to see it again. I could tell the beef-jerky-looking heap was human from its stubbed limbs (the legs and arms had burned off at the elbows and knees) and its burned-out torso, which exposed a charred backbone. We buried him, out of respect as well as hygiene, and marked his grave.

On 22 February, we relocated to OP-2, immediately across from the Al Wafrah oil field, and met up with the infantry battalion we were to support. Late that night, the ground war began for me when we crossed the border into Kuwait, while early next morning, the ground war officially began. Crossing an oil field, we ran a screen for the infantry—acting as classic cavalry, looking for the bad guys—and reported enemy positions for our infantry to engage as we advanced. From the Egg Carton, an oil-workers' camp whose roads form an egg-carton-like grid, a guide vehicle led us through a cleared channel in the mine belt into the burning Al Burqan oil field. Behind us, the afternoon sun shone brightly; but in front—reminiscent of Dante's Inferno—raging oil-well fires burned, pumping acrid, oily smoke into the air and burning so hot my mustache singed. Once within that petrol pandemonium, we made contact with the enemy and all hell broke loose. People began firing weapons, tracer rounds streaked through the smoke, and we began taking scores of prisoners, while all around us the high-pressure, putrid, oil-well fires screamed deafeningly.

Because the oil pipelines channelized us onto the road, our advance toward Kuwait City was along a major road; bad for us, good for an enemy defense. Suddenly, our lead platoon spotted three T-54 tanks just off the road about 250 meters ahead. Guys began screaming over the radio, "We got tanks! We got tanks!" and green and red tracer rounds began flying back and forth. Some people shouted orders, and others just screamed, "We need help! We need help!" The heat from the fires rendered infrared scopes useless, and night-vision goggles (NVGs) did not work because the oleaginous smoke blocked out all light save the fires, which bled out anything visible with NVGs.

In the chaos, our CO called for our TOWs, but the TOW vehicle, behind me, could not maneuver for a good angle on the tanks, since we stood between it and the T-54s. Hearing the report of a TOW behind me, I jerked my head around and saw a glowing red dot—the fiery halo from the missile's rear rocket motor—coming straight for my forehead. Terrified, I knew I was about to die. But the missile flew right by me. The TOW operator, knowing he had no clear shot, guided the missile along the road close to our vehicles and, clearing the lead LAV, walked it back on target and blew up a tank. The residual TOW wire connecting the missile to the operator's controls draped harmlessly over our vehicle. He did that twice, killing two tanks.

Our lead platoon's LAV, now having a good angle on the third tank, opened fire with its M-242 Bushmaster chain gun, a 190-pound automatic weapon that fires 25mm high-explosive and armor-piercing rounds. Because the Iraqis imprudently failed to remove a spare fifty-gallon road-march fuel drum from their tank—for obvious reasons doctrine dictates dropping surplus fuel tanks before combat—the chain-gun rounds hit the drum, exploding the fuel inside. The tank's crew, baling out of the burning tank, was dispatched in a hail of chain-gun and small-arms fire, and we continued our advance.

Though now close to Kuwait City, we received orders to stop advancing, so we effected a standard cavalry maneuver—driving in a circle. Without warning, a truck fleeing the oil field trying to make its way to Kuwait City loaded with documents and maps broke into our position, unaware that it had done so until too late. Adrenaline pumping, I raised my M-16A2 rifle and, together with my executive officer and artillery officer, fired three rounds apiece into the truck. One or more of our rounds found the driver, killing him. One of the passengers took a round across his shoulder blades, barely skinning him as he dove through the space that moments ago contained a windshield, while the other took a .223 round in a buttock. We ran to the truck, rifles trained on the surviving Iraqis. Forcing them to the ground, we disarmed and handcuffed them with plastic flexi-cuffs. Next day, I spent some time with them. I gave them cigarettes and, having a smoke with them—and I don't know why I did this—told one who spoke English, "Hey, pal. Sorry we had to shoot you guys." Looking at me, he said, "Its OK. I'd have killed you if I had the chance. You did what you had to do."

From the heart of the Al Burqan, we advanced to the "traffic circle"—the oil-field headquarters area where the oil-field roads merge—and onto a two-lane hardball highway leading toward Kuwait

City. Driving north, we suddenly found ourselves surrounded on three sides by a dug-in Iraqi mechanized infantry battalion. The battalion was equipped with Chinese armored personnel carriers (PRC-50), armed with heavy machine guns. Our guys let go with chain guns, and they returned fire with heavy machine guns; while our dismounted scouts engaged them with M-16s, we began taking mortar fire. I called in our position and the relative Iraqi positions to an OV-10 Bronco— a twin-turboprop, light attack aircraft used by Marine observation squadrons—and the Bronco started calling out and marking Iraqi positions with white phosphorus rockets, the rockets' brilliant-white explosive clouds marking targets for us, easily visible even in the afternoon desert sun.

After fifteen or twenty minutes, the shooting just stopped. White flags and raised hands suddenly appeared, and scores of Iraqi soldiers surrendered en masse. Just then, a Marine F/A-18 Hornet, monitoring our frequency, thinking he was coming to our rescue, broke in on my frequency. "I understand you've got a company of Marines surrounded by an Iraqi battalion; where do you want the bombs?" Radioing back, the OV-10 pilot said, "No, no, no. Marines are surrounded but the Iraqis are surrendering." The F/A-18 pilot, violating military radio procedure, responded classically, "Ah, shit."

Though we'd taken about 150 prisoners, the rest of the battalion did not give up. Still, the immediate danger had ended and, during field interrogations, we asked them, "You were shooting us up pretty good. Why'd you stop?" They explained that, while those who surrendered were regular army, a contingent of elite Republican Guard attached to their battalion had engaged us to draw our fire and force the Iraqi regulars to fight.

Inquiring further, we asked, "Why'd you stop?"

"We killed them so we could surrender."

While the brunt of the fighting had ended for the moment, we still took mortar fire. Interrogating an English-speaking Iraqi major, I gave him cigarettes and we showed each other pictures of our kids. Seeing this put him at ease, I presented a map and asked the location of his mortarmen, and he told me. Next day, a Navy corpsman reported that the major died of a heart attack during the night. I don't know if it was anxiety from being taken prisoner, or guilt from giving up his own guys, but the poor SOB just died of a heart attack.

Ironically, we had more prisoners than Marines, all guarded only by our first sergeant and a couple of lance corporals. It was curious to observe the typical reaction when an Iraqi first learned he'd surrendered to Marines, rather than the Army. Invariably, their faces showed mixed shock and terror; they'd been taught Marines are clinically insane cannibals who, as a condition to admission, must kill an immediate-family member. But we treated them so well—providing warm meals, plenty of water, blankets, and cigarettes—that some began turning down food and smokes, having overeaten and smoked themselves sick.

That night, the wind shifted and brought back the smoke, and the Iraqis by now discerned they were up against only a company. So, between the smoke and their numerical superiority, they probably figured taking us would be a piece of cake. They figured wrong. I radioed the battalion air officer requesting air support, and he gave me three A-6E Intruders. Because the smoke precluded visual or laser fire direction, however, I had to use a radar beacon. Since we were very close to the enemy and—for whatever reason—in FAC School my only exposure to radar-beacon fire direction was in the classroom, I was scared shitless. I gave the lead Intruder our position and the relative Iraqi positions and told my CO that one minute before the attack he must pull his lead platoon back five hundred meters.

Having determined the location of the Iraqi forward line and probable assembly area and line-of-retreat, I directed eleven 500-pound bombs across the forward edge of the battle area. The concussions pelted our lead platoon with rocks and shook the ground beneath; we were so close there was no flash-to-bang time, only a flash and bang immediately after the low-flying jets roared by. The prisoners had no clue the sortie was coming and, hearing our jets overhead, and then the mass of explosions, thought we were the target and nearly rioted, clawing the sand to dig themselves in. A few more sorties, and I directed forty-four 500-pounders across the Iraqi assembly area and line-of-retreat. Then, silence.

Next morning, approaching the target area, I saw the bombs had destroyed six vehicles, severely damaged several buildings, and killed and injured scores of people; bodies and body parts littered the area. About one hundred woebegone guys left alive just stood there, hands in the air. The night before, after the bombing, I had an AC-130H Spectre gunship—a C-130 transport plane modified with side-mounted cannon and guns to provide low- and slow-flying ground support—available for "mop-up" if I wanted. Nothing would have lived through an attack by Spectre, whose M-61A1 Vulcans— 20mm six-barrel Gatling autocannons that fire at a cyclic rate of sixty-six hundred rounds per minute—can take out a football field–size area in seconds. At that point, though, since it was clear they had no fight left in them, I chose to not call in the gunship. It would have been, quite literally, overkill.

Notwithstanding that we won this battle, I learned a lesson. I'd had the chance to take out the battalion the day before but didn't, and paid for it that night. It could have been fatal; had I screwed up the beacon-tracking mission, I could have killed my own people. I ought to have called in the F/A-18 when I'd had the chance, engaging them at my convenience, not theirs. The lesson garnered is, when the opportunity presents itself, take out your enemy. He won't respect reticence; the battle will be fought later, and with no guarantee of a favorable outcome.

That morning, a pickup truck of guys from the battalion we engaged the night before tried to escape. Though we assaulted the truck with machine-gun fire, we only wounded the driver, and it was the damnedest thing I ever saw. The bullets riddled the pickup and in effect skewered the driver—three rounds penetrated the door, one each entering and exiting his left and right biceps, the tops of his left and right thighs (without hitting the femur), and his left and right calves. He somehow opened the door and hobbled out of the pickup, arms out—but not quite up—moaning in pain the little English he knew, "My name is George. I am a Christian. Don't shoot me!"

That afternoon we started the much-anticipated advance into Kuwait City. That night, 27 February, we took up a position just outside the Kuwait international airport. At first light next morning, Alpha and Charlie Companies recaptured the airfield. A Marine from my company—I don't know who—pulled down the Iraqi flag flying in front of base operations, and we raised a Kuwaiti and U.S. flag that I had brought along in my ALICE pack. After that, things started happening fast and furious, generals started showing up, then the press, and then it was over. We couldn't believe it at first. But the announcement was confirmed; the war was over.

Though a brutal reality I'd rather not have had to experience, I am proud of having fought alongside the outstanding Marines with whom I served. I never had dreams about the war, but for years I thought about it daily. I discussed it with my confessor, and I've made peace with my Maker. Like every other Marine, soldier, airman, and sailor, I did what I had to do, because it had to be done by someone.

•••

BIOGRAPHY: *Paul Michael Wojcik was born October 31, 1955, in San Diego, California. He joined the Army out of high school, serving three years. After graduating from Western Connecticut State University in 1982, he was commissioned a Marine officer and in 1984 graduated from flight school at NAS Pensacola. Now retired from the Corps, Wojcik works for the State of North Carolina as the Admin and Safety officer at Vocational Rehabilitation. He lives with his wife, Donna, and three daughters in the mountains of western North Carolina.*

Always Faithful

—By Colonel Thaddeus Paul Wojcik, Sr., USMC (ret.)—
as told to Paul Michael Wojcik

My first combat-duty assignment in World War II was at Guadalcanal, after the Allies had taken the airfield there from the Japanese on 7 August 1942. I was a Marine second lieutenant assigned to VMO-251, trained to fly the Grumman F4F-3P "Wildcat." Though well-armed and well-armored, the Wildcat nevertheless proved inferior in maneuverability and other performance measures to the Japanese fighters.

Though VMO-251 was a reconnaissance squadron, we actually trained and operated as a fighter squadron. My first combat flight involved providing cover for dive bombers in an attack on an airfield the Japanese were constructing at Munda Point on the island of New Georgia, about 170 miles northwest of Guadalcanal. I exited the ready room after the mission briefing and walked into the predawn darkness with my squadron toward the airfield.

As I seated myself in the cockpit of my plane, a current of energy coursed throughout my body and mind. Though both excited and nervous, I set aside my thoughts and focused on the tasks at hand. Engine running, I taxied down the flare-lit runway, gripping the stick with a gloved, sweaty palm and easing it forward to achieve takeoff speed. I raced down the pockmarked airstrip and lifted off.

I felt the Grumman's seven thousand pounds lift reluctantly into the darkness, leaving airfield and beach and jungle behind. Once airborne, I pulled up my wheels and turned my attention to making a good rendezvous with my squadron and testing my wing-mounted machine guns. After charging my weapons, I fired an abbreviated fusillade into the empty sky. The two bore-sighted .50 cals rattled over the roar of the engine. The muzzles erupted. Four ribbons of phosphorus-tipped tracer rounds pierced the night. The incandescent paths converged, crisscrossing about seven hundred feet in front to fall harmlessly into the dark water far ahead. They worked.

After making a good rendezvous, together with the flights of other fighters and bombers, each at its mission-determined altitude, we headed toward New Georgia. About ninety minutes later, we arrived. My first taste of combat was a furious foray into the surreal, as adrenaline arrested fear, time, and fatigue. Dive bombers screamed down in near-vertical dives, delivered their payloads from release altitudes of two thousand or even fifteen hundred feet, then quickly pulled safely up and out of their dives. The airfield below erupted in brilliant, torrid explosions.

Zeros emerged below from under camouflage netting and bowed palm trees and climbed quickly into the morning sky to enter the deadly aerobatic dance. We engaged the Zeros in an internecine merry-go-round in the air, flying round and round, the sky painted by a weave of tracer rounds. Our Grummans could take heavy punishment—the one advantage the Wildcat held over the faster, more maneuverable Zero. The Zeros that we hit did not typically fare so well. We strafed ground positions, too. Zooming fast and low over the airfield, we targeted grounded planes, refueling trucks, fuel depots, gun positions, personnel.

Finally, when it was time to head home, I realized I had become separated from my squadron.

I tried making radio contact. Silence. I dipped my portside wing and banked my plane around sharply, heading back down the slot on our predetermined route home. As my adrenaline subsided, my combat-tensed muscles relaxed and began shaking like Jell-O.

Alone, ammo pans empty, low on fuel, no radio contact. This did not bode well. I scanned the skies above, looking especially for any Bogeys that might appear, suddenly diving out from a cloud. Nothing. Behind. Nothing. Below. Nothing. Ahead. Nothing.

I continued flying and scanning the skies. My muscles stopped quivering. The roar of my Pratt & Whitney–driven propeller did nothing to silence my small, inner voice of unease. I tried to ignore it. Though concerned about being alone and weaponless in enemy-dominated skies, I did take comfort in the knowledge that my Wildcat was one helluva tough bird; guys had come back from combat with their planes pretty well shot up. Its ruggedness had even earned the Grumman Aircraft Company the moniker "Grumman Iron Works." Still, not being able to outclimb, outrun, or outmaneuver my enemy was no small issue. I grimaced, thinking of my now-innocuous machine guns. I shook my head to clear the doubts, reminded myself of the factors in my favor—my training, the heavy armor protecting my plane, the impressive record we were building in spite of the enemy's technical air superiority, that I was a United States Marine—and focused on flying and scanning the skies.

After a time, I suddenly saw ahead in the distance a glint of sunlight. I grinned. "There they are!" I thought aloud. "Yes!" I'd catch up to the other planes and head safely back to Henderson Field in good company.

Soon, though, I realized I was catching up to but a single plane. I strained my eyes looking for some sign of others. I looked above and below. Nothing. I noted I was catching up much faster than I'd have expected. Faster than I had a right to expect, in fact. "Why?" I asked myself. I peered ahead, squinting. Then, I confirmed what I hadn't wanted even to consider: the silhouette of the plane ahead was not that of a Grumman. The closely cropped hairs on the back of my neck prickled and my knuckles, set fast on the control stick, clamped down vicelike, surely turning white under my gloves. My forehead became moist with beads of sweat, and my eyes momentarily narrowed to slits as I identified the plane, a Zero. And it was flying right toward me.

So, out of ammo and unable to establish radio contact, I was flying head-on toward a Japanese fighter. Even if I could have outrun him, I could not exactly turn around. "Where would I go?" I thought. "Back to New Georgia?" My thoughts came fast and furious. His lightweight aircraft normally would be all but defenseless against my .50-cal machine guns. But, my guns were empty. I was heading toward him and had nowhere to land. If I sought cover in the clouds, he'd intercept me before I got there. And, as good and well-trained a pilot as I was, I was still a "butter-bar" on my first combat mission and had no idea who this other pilot was; he could have been Japan's top ace, for all I knew. Probably had ammunition, too.

I began to wonder what he might do. Attack me head-on, shooting me directly through my windscreen? Or pull up, then come at me from above? I continued to head straight toward him, a brazen leatherneck pilot in a bird that could take whatever punishment he might have, as though planning to shoot him right through his windscreen. I was playing chicken, as it were, in a World War II fighter plane over the South Pacific against a deadly enemy.

I kept looking for planes from my squadron. Nothing. No other planes in the skies. Good for me that he was alone; bad for me that I was alone.

I no longer noticed the sound of the 1,200-horsepower engine propelling me forward toward certain, one-sided combat. I fought to concentrate, keeping my emotions steady, trying in vain not to think of Marian, my wife, or our first child we were expecting.

He had to have seen me by now, of course, identified me as his American enemy. But, though he wasn't turning tail and running, neither was he taking a position from which to attack me from above. He would know he could outrun and outmaneuver my plane, and that my plane had the armor to sustain all but the most precise and heaviest of salvos, and (as far as he knew) the armament to bring him down with little more than a second or two of a well-directed burst from my machine guns. Still, even though he was in the better fighter plane, a one-on-one against a Wildcat would not be without risk for him. And yet he kept coming. I began sweating heavily as I realized the implications, and I prayed.

Soon we were close enough that I could make out through his windscreen the flesh tone of a face behind an oxygen mask and a pair of darkened goggles, and the white of his silk scarf against his dark flight suit.

Closer still. Time sped up.

I was now within range of his nose-mounted machine guns and wing-mounted cannon. I waited for the muzzle flashes, the lightning-bright tracer rounds streaking toward me, followed by the metalic *plink-ing* and *thud-thumping* of rounds hitting my wings or fuselage or windscreen. "Why isn't he shooting at me?" I wonder.

Every muscle in my body tensed. My vision narrowed to a tunnel through which I was flying toward an unnervingly uncertain encounter.

Closer. Then, the most bizarre event. His guns emitted no flashes; no streaks of phosphorus bridged our planes; no bullets tore through my wings or crashed into my windscreen. Time, first passing with unwelcome speed, slowed suddenly until suspended. Both of us, neither having attempted to shoot the other out of the sky, passed right by each other! To my right, I could actually see his face. I looked right at him. And he looked right back! I was close enough to identify him, had I known him. To see the bright red Rising Sun against the white silk background of his headband peeking out from under his leather helmet. To see the expression on his sun-tanned face as he looked at me, passing in slow motion.

"What is that expression he's wearing? A grin? The sunuvabitch!" He was going to come around from behind after we passed one another, I figured. He had surmised, correctly, that I was a lone wolf, defanged, and wanted to see the fear on my face before shooting me out of the sky. "Fine," I thought. I would not give him the satisfaction. No fear. And I would show him not only how formidable Grumman Iron Works could build 'em, but also how well a Marine could fly 'em.

But, it wasn't the grin of a sadist or even an expression of vengeance. It was a smile, to be sure, but a smile at once tough, amused, anxious, even chagrined. As we passed by one another, time was released from suspension when, as if on cue, we saluted each other. "Well, I'll be. . . . "

It suddenly became clear from our unspoken communiqué that the poor bastard must have run out of ammo, too! He also was alone. The last I saw his face, we were looking over our shoulders, each incredulously watching the other bound for his respective home.

As I flew on—the South Pacific below me, the azure sky all around me, and my first combat experience and that astonishing event now behind me—my consciousness suddenly grasped a certain awareness of Truth. I drew face-to-face, so to speak, with an intimate, inescapably luminescent understanding of a fundamental and undeniable reality: My life does not belong to me. The life I now possessed could be taken in an instant. And even then, only if I were lucky would I have the opportunity to see it coming first. God forbid I should die unprepared. This life that I have will end someday. I must do with it all I can as a steward of the greatest gift I could ever possess. This was an inevitably life-changing experience, one that I could never suitably describe. One that affected the way I would forever understand life and how to live it. One that added a new, even richer, meaning to the motto "Semper Fi!"

• • •

BIOGRAPHY: *Thaddeus Wojcik grew up in St. Paul, Minnesota, and worked his way through the University of Minnesota. He first enlisted in the Marines in 1940 before being commissioned, and served in the Corps for twenty-seven years, retiring at the rank of full colonel. He then returned to St. Paul and embarked on a teaching and coaching career at Hill-Murray High School. Known as the "man of one hundred stories," he was laid to rest in Arlington National Cemetery after his death on 31 October 1996.*

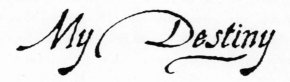

My Destiny

By Brendan Harris

When parents ask young children what they want to be when they grow up, the parents can expect answers such as "an astronaut," "a teacher," or "a firefighter," and, of course, the always-popular response, "the president of the United States." When I was posed this question as a tot, my answer was "a soldier."

Most people thought it was a stage I was going through. I loved G.I. Joe and the movie *Top Gun*. As I progressed through grade school, my teachers and parents tried desperately to entice me with different career fields and interests, but, alas, the military held its intractable hold on my interest as they slid chemistry lab or legal books in front of me. It is still true today. I can't get the military, especially the dream of becoming an officer in the United States Army, out of my head. My family attributes this single-mindedness of purpose to the TV shows and movies I watched at a young age. I disagree. My grandfathers are the ones who instilled in me the ideas of leadership through service. Their measure is what makes me yearn to protect my country.

My grandfathers are tremendous individuals. One came from steel mill country in Pennsylvania; the other from California's Central Valley. My maternal grandfather was raised an hour outside of

MY DESTINY

Pittsburgh, Pennsylvania. He enlisted in the Army to pay his way through college. He went through boot camp and eventually was given an overseas assignment in Germany. When he arrived in Germany, he was sent to the 350th Infantry Division, which was on the southern end of the East-West German border. World War II and the Korean War were recent memories at this time. The Russian Red Army was just across the border in East Germany. Barely a decade prior to my grandfather's assignment here, one of America's most famous generals, George S. Patton, was brought to a hospital in this area, where he eventually died from injuries he received in a car accident while hunting.

My grandfather finished his enlistment contract following orders and doing his duty. When this grandson was born thirty years later, he discussed with me what it is to be an American. He taught me about America's defeats and victories. "Your word is your contract," and "respect is earned," he taught me. He teaches me something in every discussion we have. When I read or view news reports regarding how people are becoming "more patriotic" because of the September 2001 terrorist attacks on our country, I am disquieted, saddened. My grandfather taught me from my earliest days that patriotism is a full-time commitment, not to be brought out for show only on certain days of the year or in times of crisis. Grandfather has always felt it is important to serve our country because it is a great country founded on beautiful principles—life, liberty, justice, and the pursuit of happiness, for all. One can serve the country for personal gain or, as my grandfather did, out of respect for the principles upon which our country was founded.

My paternal grandfather chose the military as his career. After earning his degree in criminology at Fresno State, he received his commission in the Air Force as a second lieutenant. He went to flight school, chose to fly fighters, and worked hard to do his job well. Relocating frequently with his family, he moved steadily up in rank. He served his country in Vietnam, for which he was awarded numerous medals and commendations. Eventually, he received his own fighter squadron command.

222

My grandfather's motto could easily be, "Take care of your men; if you take care of them, then they will take care of you," because he says this to me all the time. Everyone I've been able to contact who served with my grandfather concurs with that statement. He took care of the men he was charged to lead and serve. His skills as a leader, they tell me, are equal to his humanity as a man whether on the flight line or in the officers' club. One pilot who flew with him eventually went on to pilot the space shuttle; another became a four-star general and retired not too long ago as Commander of the U.S. Pacific Air Forces. From my earliest days, my grandfather was—and still is—a legend in my eyes. He taught me all about the aircraft he flew and the others he encountered. He also taught me how to get people's attention and the art of leadership. A principle of his that I use daily, whether in the classroom or on the wrestling mat, is "get the job done." I know that when the time comes, I will skillfully put into practice principles of these two personal heroes of mine.

To Bernie Hensler and Colonel Richard Harris, this grandson salutes you for giving him the best outlook and view on life any two grandfathers could ever give a young boy. It would be an honor to follow you men anytime, anywhere.

As powerful an influence as these two men have been in my life, there are others who have led me to my decision. I believe deeply in what my country stands for, the values upon which her foundation is laid. Mine is a religious family, believing deeply in God, that He has a purpose for each of us, and I believe the Lord, through His guidance through many events in life, has purposed my drive. The events of September 11, 2001, which changed America forever, reaffirmed in me the belief that someone needs to be standing a post for our magnificent country to protect her citizens from what was once unimaginable.

In the movie *Black Hawk Down*, toward the end of the film, the soldiers discuss how their friends in civilian life ask why they want to be soldiers. The number-one reason given for doing what soldiers do, is the man next to him. That's all it is. Those who serve, do so for their neighbor. General Tommy Franks recently summed up why I want to join the military when he said, "It isn't everyone who can wake up everyday and be challenged intellectually, physically, in the sense of stamina, and I like that. I can tell you it isn't for ego. And it isn't for money. It's because I like what I'm doing and I believe it's awfully important."

I will graduate high school in June 2003 and go to college that autumn. My plan is to get my degree in criminology or criminal justice while participating in the Army ROTC program, receive my commission in June of 2007, and either pursue a career in the paratroopers or go to flight school to receive helicopter training.

The following quote by the Honorable Dean Alfange, the American statesman, captures the essence of who I am: "I do not choose to be a common man. It is my right to be uncommon. I seek opportunity to develop whatever talents God gave me, not security. I do not wish to be a kept citizen, humbled and dulled by having the state look after me. I want to take a calculated risk; to dream and to build, to fail and to succeed. I refuse to barter incentive for a dole. I prefer the challenge of life to the guaranteed existence; the thrill of fulfillment to the stale calm of utopia. I will not trade freedom for beneficence or my dignity for a handout; I will never cower before any earthly master nor bend to any threat. It is my heritage to stand erect, proud and unafraid; to think and act myself, to enjoy the benefit of my creations, and to face the world boldly and say, 'This, with God's help, I have created.'"

Being a soldier will be a privilege. It has always been my destiny.

•••

BIOGRAPHY: *Brendan Harris was born in Fairfax, Virginia, in 1984. His family finally settled in Granite Bay, California, in 1997. Harris has distinguished himself as an outstanding student and wrestler in high school. He plans to attend California State University, Fresno, in the Fall of 2003, where he will study criminology and participate in Army ROTC. When he graduates, Harris will join the Army and anticipates a career within an infantry division.*

Acknowledgments

LYNNE MARIE ROMINGER:

My thanks go first to Our Lord and Savior, Jesus Christ, and the Theotokos. Without God, I am nothing and can do nothing. Next, I thank my children, Nickolaus, Sophia, Faith, and Hope, and my parents, Roberta Ann Rominger and Michael Don Rominger, for constantly supporting and helping me accomplish my dreams. Thanks must go out to my fellow "visionary," my coauthor, Milo James. A big hug and giant-sized thanks go out to my talented, hilarious, incredible students. You all amaze me each day; I've never been prouder of a group of kids than second- and third-period English 10, Fall Term 2002. I am especially proud of all the new authors—Caitlin Culbertson, Scotty Daniels, Anthony Elmer, Courtney Ferry, Melissa Hippo, Douglas Hulbert, Morgan Lo Re, Noelle Parks, Allison Rubin, Brandon Rowland, Shauna Seymour, and Chelsea Short. Thanks also to my former students who contributed, Nicholas Depner and Brendan Harris. Thank you, Mark Finlayson (at the end of this book race, you cheered me to the finish line!), Douglas Cameron, Sr., Steve Lund, Jill Labbe, Helen Scully, Amy, and Dreamy. I am also indebted to Sabina Duncan for all her help with this manuscript. I would be remiss not to thank Jennifer Basye Sander. Finally, I thank my hero, my father, Michael Don Rominger; you are the reason I first embarked on putting together this collection. Daddy, you instilled in me the necessity for character, strength, endurance, spirituality, and honor. You've saved the lives of so many and truly are one of this world's most compassionate and strong men. I love you. This book is for you.

Milo James:

With sincere gratitude I wish to acknowledge the following people in connection with writing this book: my family, without whose love, humor, and support any endeavor would be meaningless; my talented coauthor and friend, Lynne Rominger; those whose assistance and encouragement have proven invaluable in many and various ways, Julie and Victor Arreola, Rebecca Beal, Anthony Delaurentis, Sabina Duncan, Monte Engler, Peter Fields, Carla Finlayson, Mark Finlayson, Jane Garlinghouse, Tom and Patty Hartman, Sarah Hayes, Dr. Al Holtz, David Kresge, John Land, Andrea Maltese, Sam "the Man" Mancuso, Bob Messana, Jack Mudie, Pete and Mary Peterson, Sue Pinco, Robert Polich, Professor Charles Rice, Chelsea Short, Ann Sikina, Danielle Thornton, Hinga Thteen, Demetrius Volkadov, Calvin Wimbush, Christian and Dawn Word, and Michael "the Kilt" Wylie; the military and governmental liaisons from whom I sought assistance, Kacy Kossum and Lucy Lytwynsky of the Office of Public Affairs and Astronaut Office, respectively, at the Johnson Space Center; Joy White, Media Officer, Chief of Naval Education and Training; Lt. Kathleen Sandoz, USN, and YNI Sherry McKnight, USN, of the Navy Office of Information, East; 2Lt. Brandon Pollachek, USAF, of the Air Force Media Outreach Office in New York City; Capt. Michelle M. Weiss, USAF, of Air Combat Command Public Affairs; Capt. David Small, USAF, and SSgt. Robert Zoellner, USAF, of 33d Fighter Wing Public Affairs; and MSgt. Carlton Hill, USAF, of 347th Rescue Wing Public Affairs; McGuire's Irish Pub in Pensacola, Florida, for the best liverwurst and onion sandwich on the planet—I'll happily conduct future interviews amidst your lunchtime din; and the one person whom my fallibility undoubtedly caused to be unwittingly omitted from this list (mea culpa). I should also like to thank in particular Jeff and Sally Bernard, who went above and beyond the call of duty with hospitality, contacts, encouragement, intellectual intercourse, and my first sailing lesson; and, of course, Paul and Donna Wojcik, the benefit of whose friendship, interest, and support cannot be overstated.

JOINT ACKNOWLEDGMENT:

We are also, above all, indebted to the men and women whose interest in this work included recounting their personal experiences, whether through personal interviews or stories written in their own words: Don Angle; Capt. John Antedomenico, USAF; Joseph Barnard; Charles H. Brown; Frank Buday; Douglas Cameron, Sr.; Ted Cann; SSgt. (P) Scott Carmack, USAF; Robert Clark; Steven Corley, Esq.; Dr. Carlo Anthony Delaurentis, D.D.S.; John Duncan; James Elmer; Jim Fall; Mark Finlayson; "George"; Brendan Harris; Mr. "H."; Thomas Hartman; Ed Hoban; "John"; Eldon "Johnny" Johnson; Whit Johnson, CDR; Susan Kilrain, USN; "Rudy Kip"; Joseph Kraynak; David Kresge; Jill Labbe; Sanford Lebman; Wilson F. Leon; Dr. Milton Lisansky, D.D.S.; Steve Lund; LTC John H. Matthews, USA (Ret.); Chaplain (CAPT) Robert McMeekin, USAR; "Miller"; Hiro Nishimura; Jack Parks; Stephen Christopher Patterson; Lyning Moore Peterson; Robert Polich; Ed Radatz; Michael D. Rominger; Paul Eugene Rominger; Mike S.; Victor Sakellar; Ann Sikina; Bernd Simon; Marva A. Smith; Rowleen Smith; "Ted"; Jack Thompkins; James Henry Toner; Andrew Unsworth; Chaplain (LCDR) Diane Wilson, USN; Calvin Wimbush; Dr. John Witwer, M.D.; Capt. Paul Michael Wojcik, USMC (Ret.). The authors/editors particularly would like to express their gratitude to the families, and to honor the memories, of Lt. Col. Boyd Lee "Dan" Grubaugh, USAF; Warren G. Harding; Edward William Hippo; Col. Dwight R. Rowland, USAF (Ret.); Leo Scully; and Col. Thaddeus P. Wojcik, Sr., USMC (Ret.). To the students of Granite Bay High School whose exceptional work rose to a level justifying publication, we offer not merely gratitude, but also best wishes for continued success in life. Finally, but certainly not least, we would like to thank Paula Munier of Fair Winds Press (who, because of her own military heritage, intuitively understood both the vision and value of a book such as this) and Sheree Bykofsky, Janet Rosen, and Megan Buckley of Sheree Bykofsky Associates, Inc.

About the Authors

Lynne Rominger, a graduate of the University of California at Davis, lives in northern California. She is both an educator and a journalist by vocation; this is her fifth book.

Milo James, a graduate of Notre Dame Law School and Temple University, lives in New York City. James, a U.S. Army veteran, served as an intelligence analyst and Russian translator. This is his first book.